Evaluation &
Prevention
in Human Services

The *Prevention in Human Services* series:

- *Evaluation & Prevention in Human Services*, edited by Jared Hermalin and Jonathan Morell

- *Helping People to Help Themselves: Self-Help & Prevention*, edited by Leonard D. Borman, Leslie E. Borck, Robert Hess, and Frank L. Pasquale

- *Early Intervention Programs for Infants*, edited by Howard A. Moss, Robert Hess, and Carolyn Swift

- R_x *Television: Enhancing the Preventive Impact of TV*, edited by Joyce Sprafkin, Carolyn Swift, and Robert Hess

Evaluation & Prevention in Human Services

Jared Hermalin & Jonathan A. Morell,
Special Issue Editors

Volume 1, Numbers 1(1/2), Fall/Winter 1981
Prevention in Human Services

The Haworth Press
New York

Prevention in Human Services is the successor title to *Community Mental Health Review*, Volumes 1-5, 1976-1981. It is published quarterly in the Fall, Winter, Spring, and Summer.

Inquiries regarding submission of manuscripts should be directed to Robert Hess, Programs Administrator, Riverwood Community Mental Health Center, Memorial Hospital, 2681 Morton Avenue, Saint Joseph, MI 49085.

BUSINESS OFFICE. All subscription and advertising inquiries should be directed to The Haworth Press, 28 East 22 Street, New York, NY 10010. Telephone (212) 228-2800.

SUBSCRIPTIONS are on an academic year, per volume basis only. Payment must be made in U.S. or Canadian funds only. $32.00 individuals, $48.00 institutions, and $65.00 libraries. Postage and handling: U.S. orders, add $1.75; Canadian orders, add $6.00 U.S. currency or $6.50 Canadian currency. Foreign rates: individuals, add $20.00; institutions, add $30.00, libraries, add $40.00 (includes postage and handling).

CHANGE OF ADDRESS. Please notify the Subscription Department, The Haworth Press, 75 Griswold Street, Binghamton, NY 13904 of address changes. Please allow six weeks for processing; include old and new addresses, including both zip codes.

Library of Congress Cataloging in Publication Data
Main entry under title:

Evaluation & prevention in human services.

(Prevention in human services ; v. 1, no. 1/2)
Includes bibliographies.
Contents: Evaluation in prevention / Jonathan A. Morell —
Preventive intervention during the perinatal and infancy periods /
Bernard J. Shuman, Frank Masterpasqua — Federal regulations and
the lives of children in day care / Jeffrey R. Travers — [etc.]
   1. Evaluation research (Social action programs)—Addresses, essays,
lectures.   2. Social service—Evaluation—Addresses, essays, lectures.
I. Hermalin, Jared. II. Morell, Jonathan A., 1946- . III. Title: Evaluation and prevention in human services. IV. Series.

H62.E847   361.6'1'072   81-7001
ISBN 0-917724-61-5   AACR2

Evaluation & Prevention in Human Services

Prevention in Human Services
Volume 1, Numbers 1(1/2), Fall/Winter 1981

UNDERLYING MESSAGES

How do you read a journal? If you are like most readers, you probably thumb through the issue and then select and read articles related to your particular area of interest. You may skim others or read their abstracts, but unless they strike a responsive chord or you have time to kill, they go largely unread.

This first issue of *Prevention in Human Services* follows, in the main, a developmental framework which makes it easier to select particular articles. However, all of the articles should be read in their entirety because in addition to the manifest content, which may or may not be of interest, all of the articles contain underlying messages of great importance to those interested in the evaluation of prevention efforts.

Morell discusses what constitutes good evaluation, but he also reminds us that extremely complex issues and problems, which might at first seem overwhelming, can usually be addressed and solved by synthesizing and reducing them to a small number of basic concepts. His reminder is excellent and bears constant repetition.

Shuman and Masterpasqua focus on various measures and the rapidly changing infant. However, they also remind us that support for adults, the parents, is most important in ensuring the development of a healthy infant. This fits in well with findings that support is important for adults in general, especially those adults who are going through rapid changes during adult transitional periods.

Shure and Spivack describe their ICPS work and make us think of the classical tradition of science in which questions and alternative hypotheses are addressed through a series of research studies. The elegance of their systematic approach is encountered too seldom in the prevention literature.

Travers and Miller give us messages that are becoming increasingly important to prevention. The underlying message in the Travers article is that not only must the impact of services be evaluated but also the cost. Miller demonstrates that marketing research, a business concept, also occupies a significant niche in the evaluation of prevention programs. Taken together, they illus-

1

trate that prevention is a business and that in our evaluations, we must address traditional business concerns such as cost, productivity, and marketing. This is especially important given this time of limited funds and staff.

A message found in all of the articles is that evaluation of prevention activities is still very much in its infancy. If we listen closely to the overt and underlying messages in this issue and apply them to our work, we can, without a doubt, improve our evaluations and further the development of the field of prevention.

Robert Hess
Editor

INTRODUCTION

Federal, state, and local governments; funding agencies, community boards, and concerned citizen groups are increasingly demanding evidence of accountability in human services. They want proof of effective and efficient use of money and personnel, they desire assurances that programs are functioning at optimal levels, and they remain to be convinced of the necessity for further perpetuation of particular services. Given these stringent times, it is necessary that more rigorous evaluations be conducted to determine: (a) the needs of community residents, (b) their utilization and drop-out rates from service programs, (c) the quality of care being received, and (d) the costs and benefits identified with particular service components. Particularly in the field of prevention, where critics oftentimes charge that it is impossible or too difficult to evaluate the effects of given programs or services, it is most important that prevention advocates develop more sensitive assessment procedures and measurement tools to support their claims.

In this issue, we focus specifically on the evaluation of primary prevention. Utilizing a developmental framework, we consider both relevant program designs and assessment instruments demonstrated to be of value for those working in the field of primary prevention service delivery and evaluation.

Shuman and Masterpasqua's paper, "Preventive Intervention During the Perinatal and Infancy Periods: Overview and Guidelines for Evaluation," examines various measurement techniques and program protocols useful for assessing the development of children during the very early stages of life. The authors emphasize the importance of considering the physical, cognitive, social, and emotional aspects of development as part of a holistic prevention approach to enhance the development of the child.

The Travers paper, "Federal Regulations and the Lives of Children in Day Care," is based on a study contracted by the Department of Health, Education and Welfare for ascertaining types of day care programs that government should fund. Evaluation procedures were utilized to determine the relationship between staff/child ratio, group size, and staff expertise on several cognitive and behavioral outcome measures and to assess the cost-effectiveness of a variety of day care program designs. Data indicated that lower cost day care programs can be funded at no sacrifice to the child's cognitive and behavioral development. Indeed, such lower cost programs were associated with higher cognitive test scores and more positive behavioral manifestations.

Shure and Spivack's paper, "The Problem-Solving Approach to Adjustment: A Competency-Building Model of Primary Prevention," demonstrates the usefulness of a program in problem-solving techniques for managing interpersonal life situations. While discussion relates primarily to children of nursery school and kindergarten age, the approach has been shown to be effective with older age groups as well and has been adopted internationally. Of particular note is the extensive treatment given by the authors to the evaluation of both the program and research components of the study. Discussed are issues of training procedure, home and school feasibility, rater reliability, test validity, controls, and follow-up. Rigorous assessment demonstrated the problem-solving approach to be both a viable and feasible early primary prevention technique.

The final developmental paper, Miller's "Evaluation of Programs Seeking to Assist Adult Learners in Home, School and Career Transition," emphasizes the need for designing education programs for individuals entering the job market, returning to work, or changing career plans during adult life. As industrialization and automation proceed amidst a faltering economy, many people will have to find new work and develop new skills if they are to retain their well-being and financial solvency. Miller's paper aims toward evaluating the effects of one education program vis-à-vis the needs of a large, urban area. Stressed is the importance of accurate needs assessment information, nontreatment control groups, and comprehensive program effectiveness measures. Since the adult education field is relatively new, it is argued that a rigorous comparison of alternative teaching strategies is not only desirable, but necessary.

In addition to these four developmental papers, Morell presents an overview of evaluation relative to the prevention field. The paper, "Evaluation in Prevention: Implications From A General Model," focuses on the meaning of evaluation and its applicability for program planning. The issues of research validity, utility, and the role of theory in the evaluation of prevention programs are discussed in depth. Highlighted also are the special characteristics of prevention programs that the evaluator must be aware of in the formulation and design stages of a research/evaluation study.

Common to the papers are several underlying themes: (a) rigorous evaluation is necessary for demonstrating the utility of primary prevention efforts, (b) program design must be carefully tailored to meet the needs of participating target populations, (c) choice of measurement instruments should reflect a knowledge of the field (i.e., an awareness of the validity and reliability of previously constructed indices), (d) follow-up evaluations must be conducted to assess the impact of given programs over varying amounts of time, (e) control variables should be considered in study designs to guard against spurious or confounding effects, and (f) evaluators and service providers must learn to work constructively together to achieve common prevention goals. Only by coordinating and utilizing such knowledge can our hopes for the expanded success of the prevention field best be realized.

Jared Hermalin
Co-Editor, Theme Issue

EVALUATION IN PREVENTION: IMPLICATIONS FROM A GENERAL MODEL

Jonathan A. Morell

ABSTRACT. Evaluation is a many faceted, rapidly developing process which is held together by a common theme: A practical orientation toward using social programs. That practical orientation can be understood in three ways: as a total evaluation system, as a technological endeavor, or as a social research effort that has the intent of being useful as evaluation. There are three basic elements to good evaluation: validity, utility, and theory. Validity and utility must be understood in terms of specific threats to their integrity. The salience of those threats shifts with the context of evaluation activity. Theory is important because powerful evaluation designs cannot be developed, nor can results be interpreted, without an understanding of the dynamics of program action. Each aspect of evaluation—validity, utility and theory—must be considered relative to four aspects of prevention which pose particular impediments to the conduct of evaluation. Those special characteristics are: the need to mass target prevention programs, the problem of treating people who have not yet manifested symptoms, difficulties in ascertaining when prevention will be most useful, and the need to evaluate prevention programs with long term observation.

Introduction

What is evaluation? What is good evaluation? How can evaluation be used to improve prevention programs? The first two questions must be answered with general frameworks. The third is more specific and demands an exploration of two issues: What is special about prevention programs and What are the implications of those special characteristics for the conduct of evaluation? A sound treatment of these issues demands a discussion of several distinct topics.

1. a definition which shows the value of evaluation as an aid to program planning;

Please address reprint requests to Jonathan A. Morell, Hahnemann Medical College, 112 North Broad Street, Philadelphia, PA 19102.

Prevention in Human Services, Vol. 1(1/2), Fall/Winter 1981

2. threats to the validity of research;
3. threats to the utility of evaluation;
4. the role of theory in designing and interpreting evaluation studies; and
5. characteristics of prevention program which pose special challenges for evaluators.

The topic of prevention will be presented last, as general frameworks must precede specific applications. As those frameworks are presented, however, it might be useful to consider the characteristics of prevention programs which set them apart from other efforts to solve social problems. Those characteristics are:

1. the need to "mass target" prevention programs to a larger number of people than those who are actually susceptible to a problem;
2. special difficulties which arise in determining who is at risk relative to a problem which has not yet become manifest;
3. identification of periods in peoples' lives when prevention might be most effective; and
4. the extended time frames which are needed before the patterns of effects of prevention programs can be determined.

Evaluation Defined

In recent years, a large and diverse body of work has come to be known as program evaluation. The focus of these studies has ranged from explicating details of small-scale organizations to assessing the activities of multimillion dollar, multiple site programs. The methodologies have come from every field of social research and from numerous intellectual traditions (Cronbach & Associates, 1980, chap. 3; Flaherty & Morell, 1978; Freeman & Solomon, 1979; Ingle & Klauss, in press). Some of this work seems to be different from traditional forms of social science research. Much of it seems nothing more than a new label on old ways of doing things. Given all of this diversity, how might one establish a definition of evaluation which is useful for understanding the field's special capacity to generate useful information about social programs? Evaluation cannot be defined in a neat, clean, and unambiguous manner. Following the example of Roger Brown's (1965) attempt to define social psychology, evaluation will be defined here as a continually developing process which exhibits particular themes. Viewed from this perspective, it is by no means surprising that so many people do so many different things and call all of it evaluation. There are three ways to view the process of evaluation's development, each of which sheds a different light on how evaluation can help solve social problems.

Mapping the Total Evaluation System

Program evaluation is a highly focused type of applied social research the development of which can be understood in terms of seven principles.

1. Knowledge of a program's effect on its clientele is only a small part of the information that is necessary to improve that program.
2. A program does not serve all the people in a community who may benefit from its services.
3. A program or organization, by virtue of its existence, affects people and communities who are not direct recipients of the program's services.
4. The delivery of services to clientele is only part of the sum and substance of a program or an organization.
5. Programs have a need for information relative to both their effects on the "outside world" and on their internal functioning (Attkisson, Brown, & Hargreaves, 1978; Suchman, 1967).
6. The development of new forms of service is of vital concern to social programs (Morell, 1977). Further, that development can take place either within a service delivery context or outside of it.
7. The utilization of new and effective programs by service delivery organizations is not assured. There is a complex sociological dynamic which governs the adoption of innovations by organizations (Havlock, 1979; Human Interaction Research Institute, 1976).

Although no single evaluation study will embody all seven principles, those principles are manifest in the literature of the field as a whole. All seven principles and the relationships among them can be pictured schematically, as in Figure 1.

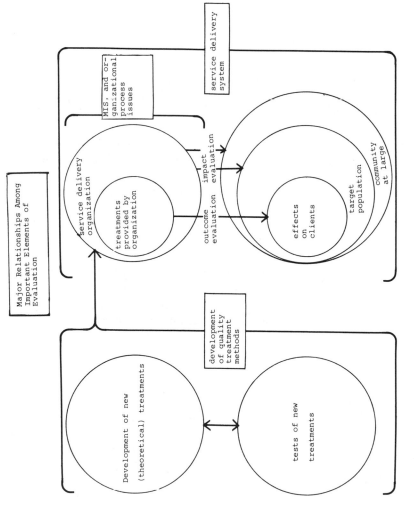

FIGURE 1. Major relationships among important elements of evaluation.

What determines where an evaluator works within this complex evaluation system? The answer is a function of the evaluator's role, work context, professional interests, and methodological leanings. It is also determined by the needs for information that are communicated to the evaluator by those to whom he or she is responsible.

Given this framework, evaluation can be defined as those research activities which take into account relationships among elements of the total evaluation system and which are oriented toward finding information which can realistically be used to improve the outcome of social programs. As an example of how this definition has tangible effects on research, consider a prevention effort in child abuse which is aimed at improving methods of identifying child-abusing parents. It is quite likely that such an effort might not be directly linked to a specific service delivery program and would very much resemble a psychological study on the prediction and explanation of behavior. In a sense, this effort belongs in the treatment development part of the diagram. Can one reasonably consider such a study to be evaluation? The evaluation like nature of the work will depend on answers to questions such as the following: Have the researchers made a point of studying indicators which, if proven successful, can easily be observed by people without highly specialized training? Do these indicators depend on data which are readily available, or is a specialized, complex, and delicate information gathering system needed? Would use of the detection system require considerable changes in the standard operating procedures of organizations that may wish to use it? Have the researchers made plans to employ research utilization principles in order to facilitate the adoption of the new procedure by service delivery organizations? People who take these questions seriously are likely to devise a study which is directly applicable to service delivery settings and which is quite different from research whose only goal is to develop as accurate as possible a technique for detecting child abusing parents.

An example can also be drawn from the part of the diagram where evaluation and programs are directly related. Imagine a study of how the consultation and education service of a community mental health center interacts with local police departments and school systems. A study of this nature could be indistinguishable from much traditional sociological research. How can duplication of effort among these organizations be reduced? What conflicts of interest impede interorganizational cooperation? What changes or new services in each organization would most help the others? None of these questions need be emphasized in a traditional sociological analysis of interorganizational relationships.

Evaluation as a Technological Endeavor

Another way to view evaluation is to see it as a primarily technological form of applied social research. (This analysis is a summary of a detailed argument presented by Morell (1979b, chap. 5). Adopting the technological perspective will affect all aspects of the research work, from initial conceptualization to final recommendations.

Rationale for program action (theory). One can find many examples of true theories which are poor guides to practical action and of untrue theories which are excellent guides to practical action (Bunge, 1966). Because scientific theories are developed primarily as guides to discovering truth, there is little reason to assume that those theories will necessarily help in the practical matter of designing effective programs. Technological theories, on the other hand, stand or fall on the basis of their practical utility. They are developed, tested, and used with that end of mind. Thus, evaluators who view programs in technological terms are much more likely to discover practically useful information than those who adopt a scientific perspective for understanding program dynamics.

Accuracy of measurement. Scientific studies must aim for as high a level of accuracy as possible, as even small discrepancies in prediction can have major implications for theory development (Ackoff, Gupta & Minas, 1962). Efforts to increase accuracy of measurement can absorb considerable resources and may detect changes which are so small as to be meaningless in uncontrolled practical settings. In technological research, the accuracy of measurement must be related to the range of detection and action that is feasible in "real world" settings.

Refutation and confirmation. The emphasis in science is on the concept of refutation, because from a logical point of view, propositions can only be proved false. (A detailed discussion of the role of refutation in science can be found in Lakatos, 1972). In technology, the emphasis is on confirmation. The goal is to raise the confidence of decision makers to a level where they will make a commitment to one course of action over another (Agassi, 1968).

Choice of problems for study. Technology and science have

fundamentally different ways of determining what should be studied. Scientific problems are well chosen if, by researching them, they are able to extend our understanding of the natural world. It may be desirable that the problem also have practical interest, but there is no logical imperative that this be the case. Technological problems are well chosen if their solution aids people who must act in practical settings. Every effort must be made to orient technological research to this end, as it is the sine qua non of technological endeavor.

Certainly, both science and technology are influenced by funding availability, by fashion, and by the personal desire of scientists and technologists to help solve social problems. In that sense, neither effort is independent of practical needs. It is also true that knowledge gained in each field is often used in the other (Bunge, 1963, 1966; Gruender, 1971). The logical differences in the two fields persist, however, and those differences are bound to affect the practical value of research. Given society's practical needs for information about programs, investment of resources in evaluation cannot be justified on the basis of potential secondary advantages of scientific research. A primarily technological perspective is required.

Intention as a Defining Characteristic of Evaluation

The concept of intention plays a crucial role in distinguishing evaluation from other forms of applied social research. At first glance, intention is an ephemeral concept that is of little practical use in deciding what is and what is not evaluation. On another level though, it is a crucial differentiator. If *evaluation intent* is carried through the work, it will have tangible consequences for many important issues. It will influence:

1. places where funding for the work is sought;
2. the organizational context where the work is carried out;
3. strategies for implementing the work;
4. researchers' perceptions of their responsibilities;
5. bodies of knowledge that are drawn upon during the course of the research;
6. how other people perceive the value of the work, and the likelihood that evaluation apprehension will arise;
7. conclusions which are drawn from the data;

8. recommendations that are made for further action;
9. the language and style of reports; and
10. ways in which study results are advertised.

Intention alone may be ephemeral, but the results of serious intention, carried through from the inception of an idea to a finished product, will greatly affect the social reality of the entire task.

Validity

Unlike other methods of helping decision makers, evaluation places major emphasis on social scientific conceptions of research validity. By so doing, evaluation has a unique capacity to increase the quality of information that is used for planning.

In dealing with the concept of validity, we shall adopt the stance that no study, however well done, can be completely trustworthy. There will always be some reason, "alternate hypothesis," that will lead us to suspect the results (Campbell & Stanley, 1966). As an example, consider an evaluation which seemed to imply that stress experienced in a population was reduced as a result of a specially constituted educational program. Did that population receive other specialized services during the time of the experimental training program? Can the improvement be explained by spontaneous recovery? Did the evaluation use trustworthy measures of stress? Can we be sure that essential elements of the program were properly implemented? Each question represents an alternate hypothesis to the claim that stress was reduced by the experimental program. Each question is based on a belief that defects in the research design—threats to validity—increase the probability that these alternate hypotheses are true.

The key to insuring validity has two elements. First, it is not necessary to dispose of all alternate hypotheses. It is only necessary to dispose of plausible threats to validity. To continue the stress example, one might cite data from previous research to show that other programs which were available to the population have no effect on stress. The second strategy is to rule out alternate hypotheses by means of research design. In the stress education example, the evaluator might have taken pains to insure a comparison group that did not receive any ancillary services while the experimental program was going on.

This paper cannot serve as a complete text on research design.

Rather, its intent is to convey an appreciation of the validity issues which must be considered in the evaluation design process and to supply a set of references where solutions to design problems can be found. To do so in a conceptually meaningful way, validity must be discussed separately for different basic types of evaluation studies. The types of evaluation presented here are used because they are helpful for understanding how major concerns about validity shift with the focus of evaluation activity. Other classifications of evaluation may be useful for other purposes. (A summary of these classifications can be found in Tripodi, Fellin, & Epstein, 1971, chap. 4). No evaluation will be a pure type, and no validity problem is exclusive to a single type of evaluation. Different evaluation types do emerge as dominant themes in evaluation studies, however, and the saliency of concerns about validity does shift with evaluation type.

Process/Organizational Evaluation

Process/organizational evaluation deals with the dynamics by which a program operates, and with the social and psychological realities of that program for the people who are associated with it. Under the rubric of this type of evaluation, one might investigate issues such as: What relationships exist among staff members? Are administrative procedures and structures adequate? What do staff members believe about their work, their organization, and the services they provide? What services are actually provided?

Because of process evaluation's focus on the structure and activity of ongoing organizations, it often involves observation and data collection during the time that program staff are actually carrying out their daily work. It may also involve a reasonable amount of interviewing of program personnel. Because of the time-consuming and often intrusive nature of such activities, there are severe limits on the amount of data which can collected. Thus, a poor data collection strategy may miss information which is crucial for protecting validity (Cannell, Lawson, & Hausser, 1975; Patton, 1980; Schatzman & Strauss, 1973).

A related problem is the evaluation apprehension which might so easily result from evaluators' appearing to check on how well people are doing their work. Such appearances, whether correct or not, might well affect what evaluators find out (Attkisson, Brown, & Hargreaves, 1978; Morell, 1977; Windle & Neigher, 1978).

Other problems arise when process evaluation is based on the analysis of data which an organization routinely collects for its own purposes. Such data are usually collected to help with management or with reporting requirements. There is no reason to assume that crucial evaluation questions can be answered with data collected for the purposes of management or accountability (Attkisson, Hargreaves, Horowitz & Sorensen, 1978; Lucas, 1975). Another difficulty is the quality of the data which may be available. Information may be missing, incorrectly recorded, or biased. Also, routinely collected data may be less precise than what is needed for effective evaluation. Access to data may also be a problem. Some computerized information systems are flexible enough to meet a wide range of needs. Other systems, however, may not be computerized at all or may store computer files in a manner that makes their flexible use difficult and expensive.

In sum, evaluators who do process/organizational studies are faced with the challenge of measuring subtle and complex aspects of an organization's behavior by means of two basic approaches, each of which places severe constraints on the amount and quality of data which may be available. If observational or interviewing approaches are used, one faces the problem of intrusiveness and of a time-consuming data collection process. These problems greatly limit the amount of information which can be collected. If existing records are used, there is the problem of drawing inference from low-quality data or from archives which may not be flexible enough for maximum evaluation utility.

Client Comparison Evaluation

Client comparison evaluation deals with the "relative effect of a program on various subpopulations of its members, between the characteristics of those who receive treatment and those who do not, or occasionally, between people who manifest a particular problem with people who do not exhibit such problems" (Morell, 1979b, p. 6). The essential character of such efforts is a study of the social and psychological factors which differentiate one group of people from another, in relation to the operation of a social program. Major validity difficulties with client comparison evaluation can be grouped under two headings: the use of psychological variables and specification of criteria for program success.

Much prevention programming is concerned with the psychological states (knowledge, attitude, belief) of a program's target population or with the relation between psychological state and behavior. Unfortunately, the use of psychological variables in evaluation poses considerable difficulty. The relation between psychological states and behavior is by no means certain. Whatever relationships do exist are subtle and are mediated by a host of factors (Mischel, 1979; Strupp & Hadley, 1977). Because of this complexity, relations between psychological states and behavior are likely to be difficult to measure in hectic service agency settings.

The choice of appropriate psychological tests is also a problem. Test development is difficult, expensive, and time consuming. Thus, there tends to be little development of tests which are tailor-made to the needs of particular evaluation situations. Tests which are already available may not have been validated on the population one is dealing with. Also, the tests may require special administration procedures which are not compatible with the pace of service delivery programs (Sellitz, Wrightsman, & Cook, 1976, chap. 6; Thorndike, 1971).

A final set of problems pertains to the need to choose tests that tap constructs which are meaningful for particular service agency settings. As an example, there is no point in telling an agency that certain types of people will not benefit from their services if the program has a funding requirement to treat those people. This requirement for practical utility greatly limits the evaluator's choice of instruments and further decreases the likelihood of developing methodologically powerful evaluation designs.

Whatever variables are chosen, they must represent a meaningful definition of who is and who is not a successful client. But what are the relevant dimensions of success, and can those dimensions be accurately measured? A search of previous research may help turn up meaningful definitions of success, but in the diverse and politicized world of social service delivery, varied opinions are bound to exist (Snapper & Seaver, in press; Patton, 1978). As an example of how difficult these questions can be, consider a client comparison study of a program aimed at decreasing recidivism among parolees. Supposing a number of the program's clients showed the following pattern of change: moderate improvement in self-image and family life, large improvement in educational skills, increased felt anxiety, and no change in criminal behavior. What decisions should the evaluator make about rating these clients on a continuum of success, and how can that rating be useful in understanding the dynamics of the program? If this question cannot be answered in a powerful manner or if any of the variables cannot be measured accurately, the conclusions of the evaluation study can be seriously compromised.

Outcome Evaluation

What happens to people when they receive a particular treatment or program? What are the immediate effects of being in such a program, as opposed to receiving no services at all or receiving other types of services? This issue is the fundamental issue in all evaluation, and its study must be a central concern in any evaluation effort (Riecken & Boruch, 1974, chap. 2).

Outcome evaluation is primarily a focused effort to draw causal inference concerning the immediate effects of a program on its clientele. The most powerful way to view outcome evaluation is by means of the research classification system set forth by Campbell & Stanley (1966) and most recently extended by Cook & Campbell (1979). The basics of the approach are defined by five assumptions.

1. All things being equal, the best evaluation method is the true experiment.
2. If true experiments cannot be done, other designs can be used which approximate true experiments to greater or lesser degrees. These approximations are called quasi-experiments.
3. All experiments and quasi-experiments are made up by varying the arrangements of four elements: groups of subjects, treatments, observations, and an allocation process for determining which subjects receive which treatments.
4. Depending on the specifics of a research situation, the same design can have more or less validity. Although all the relevant specifics cannot be stated in general, some of the more common important issues include: stability of the variables that are being studied, amount of trustworthy theory and knowledge concerning a problem under study, number of subjects which can be observed, accuracy with which measurements can be taken, and the level of analysis (psychological, behavioral, sociological, etc.) which is to be employed.
5. Appropriate research methodologies (interviewing, testing, qualitative methods, quantitative methods, etc.) are similarly context dependent (Britan, 1978).

According to the quasi-experimental approach, the art and science of methodology is to design research that is as valid as possible for a given context of study. For the sake of convenience, Cook and Campbell distinguish four types of validity. *Internal validity* refers to the trustworthiness of conclusions concerning the sample which was studied in a research setting. *External validity* is concerned with the generalizability of findings to other populations and other settings. *Statistical conclusion validity* deals with erroneous conclusions which stem from incorrect, inappropriate, or sub-optimal use of statistical tests. *Construct validity* deals with what variables, measures, or experimental manipulations are *really* about. Is the test we are using to measure health status actually measuring subjective well-being instead? Is our attempt to teach reading skills really manipulating motivation and not teaching reading skills at all? These are the types of questions which make up the problem of construct validity (Campbell & Fiske, 1959).

Outcome evaluation does not suffer from a lack of knowledge about what constitutes valid research design. Rather, problems arise from two sources (Morell, 1979b, chap. 3). First, outcome evaluation designs are delicate, i.e., small changes in the arrangements of basic elements of the research design can have major consequences for weakening validity. Second, it is often true that the more valid the basic evaluation design, the greater the likelihood that situational factors in service delivery settings will arise which will force changes in the design. This is because powerful designs often depend heavily on factors such as the random allocation of subjects to experimental conditions, the use of control groups, strict rules concerning who should receive which particular types of service, and rigid schedules for observation and measurement. They also place a premium on meticulous recording of data. Ongoing programs, however, have their own reasons for treating clients in particular ways, for deciding what kinds of people will receive what kinds of treatments, for scheduling treatment delivery, and for recording information. There is no reason to assume that the needs of programs and the needs of evaluators will coincide in these matters. Anybody who has been involved with evaluation will be able to testify that, in fact, the two sets of needs are often antithetical.

Impact Evaluation

Presumably, programs directed at individuals will also have effects that extend beyond the immediate treatment population. For example, a program which decreases the disruptive behavior of particular children in a school might have a profound effect on the learning of all the school's students, on the morale of the teachers, on the general ambiance of the school, on the relations between school and community, and on a host of other important issues.

The point of outcome evaluation is usually to determine the overall effect that a program has on its clients. There is an inherent power in such a strategy because it allows evaluators to average a program's effect over many people. By so doing, one can remove from consideration any idiosyncratic changes that may be attributable to particular individuals. Impact evaluation often cannot avail itself of this powerful strategy. In many cases, impact evaluation deals with the effect of a program not on individuals, but on other organizations or communities. As an example, one might do outcome evaluation on the effect of prenatal education on mothers and children. Impact evaluation of that program, however, may deal with the program's effect on the overall demand for social services within particular communities. The jump from mothers and children to communities greatly reduces the number of units of observation. As that number decreases, so too does the power and sensitivity of statistical analyses which may be performed.

A second problem is that impact evaluation often deals with factors which might be only tangentially affected by the program in question. To continue the previous example, the demand for social services may well be affected by a host of factors other than the prenatal program, all of which must be accounted for if the impact evaluation is to be valid.

If multiple treatment sites are used, there is the added difficulty of knowing precisely what the treatments were, as it is quite likely that different organizations implement the same program in a variety of different ways (Boruch & Gomez, 1977; Policy Studies Journal, 1980; Williams, 1976).

Follow-up Evaluation

Follow-up evaluation is evaluation that focuses on the effects of a program on people after they have left the immediate locus of treatment. What patterns of positive and negative program consequences emerge over time? How does the fact of having received a treatment enter into the fabric of a person's life? Questions of this type cannot be answered with a short term research perspective. Because delayed action effects are so important in prevention, follow-up studies must play a central role in the evaluation of those programs. Because of the difficulty and expense of face-to-face interviewing in the field, evaluators must make every effort to collect representative data by the most efficient means possible. Survey research methodologies are admirably suited to this task (Dillman, 1978; Moser & Kalton, 1972; Sudman, 1976).

Special sampling problems are bound to arise in any attempt to follow treatment recipients through time. Primarily, the issue is whether certain types of people are more easily located that others and whether there are systematic differences between those who agree to furnish data and those who do not. An important extension of this question is whether the "drop out dynamic" changes over time (Banks & Frankel, 1979; Marcus et al., 1972).

Measurement difficulties also pose serious threats to follow-up evaluation. If people are interviewed at more than one point in time as is desirable in follow-up evaluation, is there a reactivity problem? Can one trust respondents' answers to questions which require that they remember what has happened to them over a relatively long period of time? These basic measurement problems are particularly salient in the extended time frames that are needed for follow-up evaluation (Morell, 1979a).

In addition to problems of measurement bias, there is also the phenomenon of effect attenuation to contend with. Beneficial or harmful program effects may decrease because of the removal of their immediate cause, the program. New events in people's lives may push them in many different directions. Random fluctuations in measurement and in people's behavior will increasingly obscure program effects. Because of these factors, evaluators need more and more sensitive measuring instruments and larger sample size as the length of follow-up increases. ("Snowballing," and self-sustaining program effects are also possible. Unfortunately, there are all too few examples of these.)

If possible, as the length of follow-up increases, the myriad events which impact people's lives will inevitably overshadow the specific effects of a prevention program which took place at some time in the past. Thus, as the length of follow-up increases, evaluation more and more resembles research on people's life styles and becomes less and less a specific study of the effects of a particular program. Given that a researcher is studying lifestyle, with its many subtleties and nuances, how might one trace the effect of a particular life event, the treatment, as it winds its way into the fabric of a person's life? This problem goes beyond the measurement difficulties cited above. It is a question of how, with only limited opportunity for observation and a few questionnaire responses, one can tease out reasons why people act as they do in uncontrolled natural settings.

Conclusion

All research is a mixture of three themes: parameter estimation, detection of patterns of events, and efforts to draw causal inference. These themes are illustrated by the following questions: How many boarding homes patients are there in our catchment area? What types of problems do those patients tend to have? Is our intervention program effective in reducing those problems? All of the threats to validity mentioned in this section and all of the types of evaluation presented contain elements of these three basic types of research. Is measurement accurate and unbiased? Can we discern pattern from noise? Can we draw causal inference? These problems continually recur in different guises in all evaluation settings. This section has been an attempt to show how validity difficulties shift with needs for evaluation information and to convey an understanding of the challenges faced by evaluators when they try to develop valid evaluation studies.

Threats to Utility

Just as one may speak of threats to the validity of research, so may one speak about threats to the utility of evaluation. Why is evaluation not used, and what might be done about it? The key to the answer lies in understanding how information is used in decision making contexts. Once that is understood, strategies can be developed to increase the utility of information that is generated by evaluators. Those strategies must operate on two levels. First, evaluations must be designed to increase the probability that the information yielded will be useful in practical contexts. Second, the evaluator must adopt strategies for the implementation of evaluation and for the use of results, which are specifically designed to increase utilization. As with the section on validity, space will not permit a detailed description of what these strategies are. The intent here is to convey a sense of the primary concerns that must be dealt with, an understanding of when those concerns become operative, and a set of references which will allow the reader to explore these issues in greater detail.

Timing of Decision Making

Evaluators are often told that the timeliness of their information is crucial. Information can only be used if it is available before a decision is made, and while the decision-making process is still going on. But how is one to know when a decision-making process is going on, and the point at which a decision is made? Unfortunately, it is extremely difficult to make such determinations. There is a difference between the formal process of making a decision and the less overt processes by which people think, ponder, consult with each other, and act. In addition, many decisions and policies develop slowly and almost imperceptibly, as organizations function daily and have to confront many small situations which, taken together, add up to the formation of policy. The neat, clean process of weighing available evidence and forming a policy is illusory. The real process is infinitely more subtle, more complex, and less sharply defined. Carol Weiss (1980) has researched this situation extensively, and has aptly summed it up with the phrase "knowledge creep and decision accretion." Without a doubt, some times are more auspicious than others for furnishing evaluation information, but knowing when those times exist becomes a matter for considerable sensitivity and skill. Evaluators who attend only to formal decision making schedules cannot be effective.

The Reward System for Politicians

By and large, politicians get their rewards from implementing programs, not from retrospective analyses which show that old programs were successful (Brandl, 1978). By the time information is available on the success of programs, the attention of politicians, and their constituencies, has moved on to other problems. It is no small task to get a program instituted through the political process. Legislative support must be obtained. Compromises must be negotiated. The interests and needs of constituencies must be satisfied. Budgetary problems must be resolved. Hearings must often be arranged. Because the entire process is difficult and time-consuming, it is no wonder that professional and personal satisfaction derives from making programs happen. Evaluators simply cannot assume that under normal circumstances, politicians will have much use for information which indicates that functioning programs need to be changed. The most likely context for evaluation utility is when evaluation information relates to new programs or changes in old programs which are under active political consideration. Not only must the timing of the evaluation be appropriate, but the results must be applicable to the new situation which is being proposed. Not all decision makers are subject to the political reward system, but evaluators certainly meet many who are. If evaluators are not sensitive to that reward structure, evaluation utilization will most assuredly suffer.

Goals of Maintenance and Goals of Service—the Need to Target Information

Organizations have two sets of goals; those of organizational maintenance and their stated goals of service. Etzioni (1969) makes the point that both sets of goals are important, both are legitimate, and both require a share of an organization's resources. Only one set of goals, however, those of service, tend to be articulated to the public as organizational objectives. Etzioni argues that it may be impossible for organizations to meet their stated service goals because doing so would drain too many resources from the equally important persuit of maintenance goals. Etzioni completes his argument with the claim that evaluators ignore maintenance needs and tend to evaluate organizations relative to their public goals of service. The entire problem is exacerbated because exaggeration is an inherent part of stating service goals. Campbell makes the point that advocacy necessarily entails exaggeration and inflated claims (Note 1). If one considers a program's administrators and personnel as advocates for their organization, it is reasonable to assume that stated goals of service will be highly unrealistic.

If an evaluation is to be useful, it must concentrate on a reasonable mix of organizational and service goals, and it must focus on a range of accomplishments which are realistic within a program's capability.

Information as a Dysfunctional Element in Organizations

Administrators are put in a serious bind if they know that an action is called for and they also know that, because of political, economic, or other reasons, action cannot be taken. In such cases, avoidance may be the most sensible and rational tactic that an administrator can employ. Evaluators who do not recognize this problem may find themselves trying to force-feed information to people who have an accurate sense of what that information will indicate and who have good reason for not wanting to know any more.

A second problem is that organizations can only tolerate a limited amount of change. Beyond that point, any change, no matter how sensible, is dysfunctional (Wildavsky, 1972). Organizational procedures, lines of communication, mandates—all of these must have some stability if an organization is to be efficient and effective. If an evaluation threatens that stability, utilization of that evaluation will be negligible.

The Inconsistency of Goals

It is not likely that people will have a clearly articulated sense of what an organization's goals are. It is equally unlikely that all interested parties will agree on a priority order for the goals of a program. It is entirely likely that a program's goals will change as time goes on. Opinions change. Client populations change. Personnel changes. Definitions of social problems change. Why should a program's goals or the goals of those who use evaluation information remain stable? (A comprehensive analysis of the goals problem can be found in Patton, 1978, chaps. 6 & 7). If evaluators are to produce useful information, they must be able to discover program goals which are generally agreed upon and which are likely to have some stability as the program changes with time. The difficulty of obtaining this information is a major threat to the utility of evaluation.

Lack of Belief in Science

One of the most important claims made for evaluation is that it brings the power of social science to bear on the problem of understanding the actions of social programs. In a sense, the credibility of the field rests on its roots in the scientific research enterprise. But how credible is scientific evidence in the eyes of the public? We can all site examples of research which has been shown to be wrong, and we all have an intuitive sense that experience and wisdom are often more correct than the findings of scientific research. There are situations where research evidence is better than other types of information, but evaluators cannot assume that this belief will automatically be accepted. Utility is bound to suffer if that credibility is not specifically advocated.

The Role of Evaluation in Shaping Opinion

In large measure, people do not base their decisions on any single discrete piece of evidence. Rather, people are influenced by the consensus of opinion of a relatively small group of people they have come to know and trust. (I call this the "kings advisors" phenomenon). It must be so, as decision makers must strike a balance between the need to be open to information and the need to be insulated from the continual stream of conflicting opinion which assails people with power. People also base their decisions on a set of beliefs which they have built up over time and which is relatively invulnerable to discrete inputs. Thus, in large measure, the effective evaluation is one that aims at influencing a "conventional wisdom" among a group of people, rather than at providing a critical piece of information to a single decision maker. Many evaluators do not take the "climate of opinion" issue seriously, and, as a result, their work is grossly underutilized.

It is also important to realize that many factors go into the making of a decision—personal beliefs, beliefs of others, evidence that did not come from evaluation studies, economic considerations, political factors, and the like. In the practical world of management and policy, evaluation is simply one more consideration in the complex decision-making process. The utility of evaluation will increase only if evaluators understand what is competing with evaluation for influence in decision making and if they take steps to increase the influence of their work. In general, two strategies may be used to accomplish this goal. Evaluators might try to design studies which complement the types of information which are known to be influential in a given situation. Second, evaluators might use the strategies of organizational change in order to effectively advocate the use of their work (Havlock and Havlock, 1973).

Realm of Action of Decision Makers

Any social program involves a diverse group of people who stand at varying distances from the direct delivery of service to clients. As an example, teachers, principals, school board members, state and federal education officials, and legislators all fall at different places on this continuum. As one moves along the continuum, there are changes in people's job tasks, amount of money they are responsible for, number and types of constituencies they are responsible to, and, consequently, their beliefs about what constitutes a successful program. At each point on the continuum, people's realm of action changes. As that realm of action changes, so too does the need for information. Those differences include issues of subject matter, levels of analysis, models of program action, and fields of study. To continue with the school system example, consider the needs of teachers and school board members for evaluation information. Evaluators who wish to serve the vital interests of teachers might generate information based on group dynamic theories of how the classroom behavior of individual children can be changed. School board members may have a more direct interest in information based on sociological and economic models of what happens to schools under various combinations of funding, ethnic makeup, and class size. Evaluations which produce information aimed at one realm of action may be intellectually interesting to people operating in another realm of action, but of no practical utility.

Another aspect of the realm of action concept is that four general categories of evaluation utility can be discerned. Evaluation which is aimed at one type of utility may not be appropriate for other types (Morell, 1979b, chap. 4). Evaluation can be used to establish realistic expectations as to what a program can and cannot accomplish, to help those engaged in service delivery to be more effective, to aid in long range planning, and for political purposes. The following example will serve to illustrate how the entire nature of an evaluation effort may change depending on which type of utility is most desired.

Consider an evaluation of efforts to implement wide-scale teaching of first aid procedures. Evaluation based on determining realistic expectations may focus on estimations of, the number of people who can potentially be trained to acceptable levels of proficiency, the likelihood that such trainees will come in contact with appropriate emergency situations, the likelihood that trainees will actually use what they have learned, and the potential for first aid action to actually help those who are injured. Evaluation aimed at program personnel would look at the effectiveness of recruiting people for the courses, effectiveness of the teaching methods employed, the benefits of books and other teaching aids, the level of skill that students actually gained, and reasons why students failed to achieve in particular areas. Planners would most likely want to know, the number of lives saved by virtue of the training, the number of medical problems ameliorated by virtue of training, relationships among funding roles, the structure of the service delivery system, the delivery of effective training, and, the medical accuracy of the books and materials that are recommended for general use by all programs.

Each of the evaluations presented in the above example would require a major commitment of time and resources, and it is most unlikely that all the objectives mentioned above could be met in a single evaluation effort. Utility is bound to suffer if evaluators do not determine, in the design stages of their studies, which type of utility is most needed.

Summary

Each of the threats to utility presented above represents a different set of impediments to the utilization of evaluation information. A consideration of each threat will lead to specific decisions concerning each of the following questions:

— Who should be involved in the choice of an evaluation design?
— What should the design be in terms of—methodology, information collected, and models of program action?
— How should the evaluation be implemented, and who should be involved in those choices?
— What should the pace of evaluation work be?
— What idiom and what tone are appropriate for oral and written reports?
— How should one advocate for the use of the results?

Just as with validity, no threat to utility can be completely obviated. Still, there is no doubt that evaluation information is utilized (Alkin, Daillak & White, 1979; Patton, 1978, chap. 2; Weiss, 1980). If special threats to utility are dealt with as carefully as possible, the likelihood of that utilization will be further increased.

Theory

Kurt Lewin's famous dictum "there is nothing so useful as a good theory" can be thought of as a logical extension of three other principles:

— There is nothing so necessary as some theory.
— Implicit or explicit, theory is always with us.
— We may as well try to exploit the power of theory to as great a degree as possible.

As an illustration of these truths, consider the following example. An evaluator has studied the effectiveness of an outreach program designed to increase the numbers of parents who immunize their children. The evaluator has collected data on parents' knowledge about the availability of immunization programs and about the importance of immunization, on the commitment of community leaders to the immunization program, and on the increase in the number of parents who avail themselves of immunization services. The results of the evaluation indicate high levels of knowledge, medium commitment on the part of the community leaders, and moderately positive changes in immunization behavior. The program was carried out because of a high priority placed by health officials on increasing the number of immunized children.

How should these results be interpreted? Should the program increase, decrease, or maintain its educational activities? Should the program increase, decrease, or maintain its efforts to enlist the aid of community leaders? Are none of the results satisfactory, and is a radical restructuring of the program necessary? None of these questions can be answered without a theory which attempts to explain the relationships among knowledge, leader commitment, and immunization behavior. Suppose we believed that, in light of the difficulty of the problem, a reasonable amount of behavior change was effected and that both high leader involvement and high parent knowledge are crucial for behavior change. In such a case, we might conclude that the program is doing reasonably well, and that it should work at improving its liaison with community leaders. On the other hand, we might believe that the amount of behavior change was disappointing and that parent knowledge is the most important element in promoting immunization. In this case, the program has serious flaws, and must be radically restructured.

The same pattern of results has led to radically different recommendations, and all because of different theories used to guide data interpretation. The need for theory also extends beyond data interpretation strategy, as something led the evaluator to measure those variables in the first place. At all levels, the more clearly articulated the theory and the more powerful the theory, the greater the likelihood that evaluation will lead to improved social programs.

Another example shows the importance of theory as it relates to program implementation. It is axiomatic that programs as implemented are never the same as programs as designed. Consequently, it is important to understand implementation dynamics if programs are to be improved. Imagine an English as a Second Language

Program which has been carefully worked out by curriculum specialists. It is likely that the program developers would specify many aspects of service delivery. A few of these might include amount of teaching time per week, number of children per class, qualifications of instructors, a particular order for lessons and exercises, and the use of particular audiovisual aids. In addition, the program might have a basic assumption that children should be rewarded equally for cognitive and for affective learning. Finally, the program might make implicit assumptions about teacher acceptance of the program and the support of administrators for its use. Two things are certain: first, that the program as implemented will be different from the experimental program as it was developed, and second, that the evaluator will not have the resources to accurately measure all of the factors mentioned above. Which ones should be measured? Once measured, how should the information be interpreted to help understand the program's successes and failures? Without a theory of program implementation, those choices cannot be made. If the theory is weak or not well specified, relatively poor choices will probably be made.

Finally, one can draw examples of more general theories that may be employed. Consider a job training program designed to remove people from the need to receive welfare. Over and above evaluating the actual success of skill training, one might choose a wide variety of factors to help explain the program's successes and failures and to point ways for improving the program. Personality factors of participants might be included—intelligence, motivation, ability to cope with stress, need achievement, locus of control, past work experience, and education. Social support factors might also be studied—family living arrangements, support of family for the worker's changed life style, and the like. One might look at institutional factors such as the nature of the work setting and its compatibility with the cultural background of the worker.

It is not enough to argue that all of these factors may be important and that they should all be measured. Resources are limited and choices must be made. Even if each dimension were represented, some would be much better documented than others. In addition, merely collecting all the data would not help when it came time to formulate an analysis plan, to interpret the findings, and to make recommendations. Having all the information would not help at that point. At some point in the analysis, choices would have to be made as to what factors to relate to others, and the meaning for the program of any patterns which were observed would have to be interpreted. None of that can be done without the use of theory.

These examples illustrate the centrality of theory as a guiding force in the evaluation of prevention programs. That emphasis on theory is not unique to the evaluation of prevention. Rather, it is based on strong traditions, both in the general evaluation literature and in philosophy. The general point in these writings is that without the guidance of theory, data alone cannot provide meaningful explanations of events (Bruner, 1957; Kaplan, 1964, chap. 8; Riecken, 1972; Weiss, 1972; Campbell, Note 2). The overall lesson is that data must be embedded in a conceptual framework if it is to be interpreted in a meaningful way.

Theory need not be esoteric, complex, or difficult to understand. It might be complex and difficult, but that depends on what is needed to explain a phenomenon of interest. It is certainly desirable to keep theory as simple as possible. It is most assuredly necessary to make theory as powerful as possible. To that end, all available knowledge, experience, and wisdom should be brought to bear. In some cases, already existing theories can be used to guide evaluation. In other cases, "local" theories must be derived to meet particular needs. Whatever is most useful is what should be done. That is the only rule.

Evaluation and Prevention

Because prevention efforts span every type of social programming, it is no small effort to determine those characteristics which prevention programs have in common and which set them apart from other efforts to solve social problems. Four such characteristics can be identified: mass targeting of services, at-risk determination, identification of the most auspicious times for prevention treatment, and the need for long range perspectives in prevention programs. All of these issues may be important for any social program; the difference is one of relative emphasis. In prevention programs, these issues are central and conceptually important concerns which must be given high priority. That priority must be reflected in the work of evaluators, and doing so poses special problems for the design of powerful evaluation studies. It is also true that prevention programs share many evaluation concerns in common with other types of social programs. Evaluation can and should deal with these issues, and the general framework presented in this paper can be used for that purpose, but prevention programs are special, and I hope to show how those special characteristics must be treated if meaningful evaluation of prevention efforts is to be carried out.

It would be too long and tedious to show how the special characteristics of prevention relate to each nook and cranny of the general evaluation framework which has been presented so far. Specific examples can be presented, however, and these will serve to illustrate general case.

Mass Targeting

Prevention programs, almost by necessity, tend to be aimed at relatively large populations. It must be so, as the number of people susceptible to a problem is certain to exceed the number of people who will actually exhibit that problem. In addition, prudence argues for a liberal interpretation of who is at risk. Both of these factors lead to the extension of prevention services to a relatively large number of people.

Because mass targeting is often so important in prevention programming, evaluators must pay special attention to the effectiveness of those efforts. Call it outreach or advertising, it is a crucial aspect of prevention, and its effectiveness must be determined.

Theory. When evaluating the impact of an outreach effort, which audience should receive the most attention—potential participants, their social support networks, or their authority structures? What aspects of advertising are important—timing, content, form, or frequency? Are the messages conveyed by the outreach effort credible and salient? If so, what situational and logistic factors might influence whether people act on the basis of those messages? In sum, what are the dynamics by which an outreach effort produces clients for a prevention program? Choices must be made as to what those operative elements are, as no single evaluation can be all encompassing. Those choices inevitably reflect theories of how outreach efforts relate to the reasons why people avail themselves of prevention services.

Validity. How might one determine the effect of an advertising effort on the beliefs and actions of an audience? Ideally, this question should be answered by setting up specially constituted test groups which are representative of the target population and by systematically varying the type and amount of information which they receive. With this information as a base, various field tests should then be carried out. In practical evaluation settings, there is seldom the time, money, or resources to conduct such a study. As a far inferior alternative, evaluators are forced to assess uncontrolled outreach efforts. The major problem is such a strategy is that it forces the evaluator to answer three research questions simultaneously and in a setting that does not allow observation of the effect of each question on the others. At the same time and in the same setting, the evaluator must determine the value of the content of the advertising, the amount of advertising that reached people, and the influence of that advertising on various types of people. In such a case, it is extremely difficult to answer any of these questions particularly well.

Utility. A major use of evaluation is to help people develop realistic expectations as to what a program can and cannot accomplish. This is a need which affects almost all people concerned with a program, across all realms of action which decision makers may have. Determining realistic expectations in prevention programs is confounded by the fact that two different effectiveness estimates can be made. First, one might measure effectiveness relative to an entire target population, a number which is deliberately made larger than the number of people who may actually benefit from a program. Second, one can determine which subset of a target population is actually susceptible to a problem and estimate effectiveness relative to that second group. Unfortunately, the nature of prevention does not admit simple observation as a means of determining whether a person is susceptible to program intervention, hence, the need for mass targeting and for unknown discrepancies between a program's target audience and the pool of people who can actually be helped. That unknown discrepancy makes it extremely difficult for evaluators to realistically estimate what a program might be able to accomplish.

Risk Determination

Efficiency and a commitment to delivering appropriate services demand efforts to identify people most in need of service. This can be accomplished by the use of either demographic or individual characteristics of potential candidates for a program. Demographic information tends to involve gross categories which are necessarily imprecise indicators of who is at risk. Assessment of individual characteristics involves case by case scrutiny of potential service recipients and is necessarily labor intensive. Thus, the effective and efficient determination of high-risk populations is a difficult and problematic issue in prevention programming. Even with the most effective targeting system, prevention recipients will differ in their likelihood of manifesting an as yet unseen problem. This issue can be seen to operate across all aspects of evaluation concern—theory, validity, and utility.

Theory.   Given that one is dealing with a high-risk population, how might one differentiate those with relatively higher and lower risk of exhibiting a problem? Such determinations are particularly difficult because the initial determination of high risk may have already been made on the basis of the best information that is easily available. Cutting the risk determination even more finely is not likely to be easy or inexpensive. Such determinations are important, however, because of the need to effectively allocate resources and because much valuable information can be gained by studying the relative effectiveness of a program on higher and lower risk individuals. In making such determinations, evaluators have a choice of several general classes of variables: personal characteristics of treatment recipients, social support factors, stress factors in the environment, and the like. Data is often lacking to guide such choices, and theory, a model of program action, must substitute for empirical knowledge as to which factors will most clearly distinguish fine gradations of relative risk.

Validity.   If an evaluation is to yield data on program effectiveness as a function of risk, the evaluator must assess intermediate and mediating variables which may lead to the overt manifestation of the problem. These variables may be social or psychological, but they will almost certainly be difficult to measure in valid and reliable ways. Even if proper measurements could be made, powerful research designs will necessitate using those measures as criteria to determine how the program should treat its clients. It will be hard enough for an evaluator to employ those measures merely as an assessment device. It will be harder still to use them as a treatment allocation method in a service delivery setting.

Utility.   Many prevention programs are aimed at populations which are thought, correctly, to have a relatively high risk of exhibiting a problem. Further, many prevention programs are good things in and of themselves, regardless of their relative preventive effects. As an example, who would argue that compensatory education programs are not a good idea for disadvantaged children? Further, many people have strong personal beliefs concerning who is at risk and who should receive treatment. Evaluation, on the other hand, attempts to make a rigorous determination of who is at risk and of who can be helped. Such an attempt may well come up with results which are counterintuitive, or which would exclude many people from a program. In cases where evaluation and cherished beliefs conflict, an evaluator's audience is more likely to question the power of science than give up their cherished beliefs. This problem is particularly difficult in prevention programming because people have strong beliefs about who is at risk and because the nature of prevention precludes using actual problem manifestation as a criteria for acceptance into a program.

Timing of Treatment Administration

Assuming that a person will exhibit a particular problem, when in that person's life will preventive treatment have the most impact? Just as it is important to understand a prevention program's effect on different types of people, so is it necessary to ascertain whether prevention efforts are differentially effective at different times in people's lives. The difficulties presented by this need are analogous to those dealt with in the previous section. There is an added difficulty, however, because it now becomes necessary to trace variations in risk not only across individuals, but within the lives of individuals as well. Thus, theory must be extended to explain how risk varies within individuals. Valid evaluation designs must assess program impact relative to fluctuations in a person's susceptibility to treatment. Useful evaluation must counter intuitive beliefs, not only about types of people who may need prevention services, but it must also deal with beliefs about when treatments will be effective. The need to deal with differences both within and among people seriously complicates efforts to produce evaluation which is both useful and valid. Research designs must account for inter- and intra-individual differences. Threats to utility are similarly complicated, as is the need to develop or discover suitable theoretical structures and models of program action.

Extended Time Frames

There are four reasons why extended time frames are crucial for assessing the effectiveness of prevention programs. First, one cannot predict precisely when a problem will emerge. Second, prevention programs have a short duration relative to the time span when a problem may emerge. Thus, it often does not make sense to evaluate prevention programs in terms of immediate postprogram effects. Third, it is reasonable to assume that positive or negative effects of a prevention program will be observable only some time after the program has taken place. Finally, it is likely that the effects of a prevention program will fluctuate over time and that different effects may change in different ways.

Theory   People's willingness to cooperate with evaluators may well decrease as the length of time after completion of a program increases. Unfortunately, the need for precise and detailed evaluation information may increase with the length of follow-up. This is because the relationship between a prevention effort and a person's life-style may become more complex and subtle as program effects weave themselves into the warp and woof of a person's life. Thus, the need for data increases at precisely the same time as when the availability of that data is likely to decrease. Because of these conflicting trends, evaluators must be as efficient as possible when deciding what questions to ask their respondents. What data will be most helpful in explaining a highly complex social phenomenon? A well developed theory of program action is crucial in making such determinations.

Validity.   No matter how clever one is in the use of theory, information needs will be many, data collection opportunities will be few, and the quality of evaluation is bound to suffer. Further, the problem of nonresponse and of differential nonresponse across different treatment groups is likely to get worse as the length of follow-up increases.

Utility.   The need for extended time frames raises serious problems of balance between evaluation's emphasis on goals of service relative to goals of program maintenance. It is a problem that touches on several important aspects of utility, most notably, varying realms of action for different decision makers and political uses of evaluation. Goals of organizational maintenance require that program administrators have some type of useful information when it becomes necessary to defend their programs and to apply for further funding. Where immediate positive outcomes are possible, goals of organizational maintenance may well fit with evaluation of service goals, as positive program effects can be used to secure further funding. This is not likely in the case of prevention programs, however, because immediate positive effects are not likely or may be of only secondary interest to funders. The problem might be solved if appropriate intermediate factors leading to long term prevention could be included in the evaluation study, but such a requirement imposes the need to find such factors, to measure them accurately, and to convince various constituencies that those variables are, in fact, related to long term prevention. It may well be possible to accomplish these tasks, but doing so imposes a difficult and delicate task on the evaluator.

Summary

Four issues tend to be more important for prevention programs than for other types of social programs. First, prevention programs must target services for considerably more people than are actually in need of those services. The need for such a strategy stems from the difficulty of knowing in advance who will manifest a particular difficulty or symptom. Second, prevention programs must carefully assess the likelihood that people will manifest a problem. Mass targeting notwithstanding, efficiency and economy dictate that some attempt be made to selectively treat those who most need treatment. Third, the timing of treatment is important, again, because of the unknowns involved in preventing not yet overt problems. It is reasonable to assume that some periods in people's lives are more auspicious than others for the application of some prevention efforts. Finally, prevention efforts must be evaluated with long range perspectives, as the nature of prevention implies that many consequences of a program will not be manifested until some time after a treatment has been applied.

Although any of these concerns might be present in a wide variety of social programs, the importance attached to them is likely to be particularly high in the case of prevention. That priority must be reflected in the efforts of evaluators, who must pay special attention to the practical and conceptual difficulties encountered in attempts to evaluate programs relative to these four program characteristics.

REFERENCE NOTES

1. Campbell, D. T. *Methods for the experimenting society*. Unpublished manuscript, Maxwell School, Syracuse University, 1971.
2. Campbell, D. T. *Qualitative knowing in action research*. Kurt Lewin Memorial Address, Society for the Psychological Study of Social Issues, Meeting of the American Psychological Association, New Orleans, 1974.

REFERENCES

Ackoff, R. L, Gupta, S. K., & Minas, S. *Scientific method: Optimizing applied research designs*. New York: Wiley, 1962.
Agassi, J. The logic of technological development. *Proceedings of the XIV International Congress of Philosophy*, Vienna, 1968, 383–388.

Alkin, M. C., Daillak, R., & White, P. *Using evaluations: Does evaluation make a difference?* Beverly Hills, CA: Sage Publications, 1979.
Attkisson, C. C., Brown, T. R., & Hargreaves, W. A. Roles and functions of evaluation in human service programs. In C. C. Attkisson, W. A. Hargreaves, M. J. Horowitz, J. E. Sorensen (Eds.), *Evaluation of human service programs.* New York: Academic Press, 1978.
Attkisson, D. C., Hargreaves, W. A., Horowitz, M. J., & Sorensen, J. E. (Eds.). *Evaluation of human service programs.* New York: Academic Press, 1978.
Banks, M. J., & Frankel, M. R. Adjusting for total nonresponse. In R. Andersen, J. Kasper, & M. R. Frankel (Eds.), *Total survey error.* San Francisco: Jossey-Bass, 1979.
Boruch, R. F., & Gomez, H. Sensitivity, impact and theory in impact evaluation. *Professional Psychology*, 1977, *8*, 411–434.
Brandl, J. E. Evaluation and politics. *Evaluation*, 1978, special issue, 6–7.
Britan, G. M. Experimental and contextual models of program evaluation. *Evaluation and Program Planning*, 1978, *1*, 229–234.
Brown, R. *Social psychology.* New York: The Free Press, 1965.
Bruner, J. S. Going beyond the information given. In J. S. Bruner et al. (Eds.), *Contemporary approaches to cognition.* Cambridge, MA: Harvard University Press, 1957.
Bunge, M. *The myth of simplicity: Problems of scientific philosophy.* Englewood Cliffs, NJ: Prentice-Hall, 1963.
Bunge, M. Technology as applied science. *Technology and Culture*, 1966, *7*, 329–347.
Campbell, D. T., & Fiske, D. W. Convergent and discriminant validation by the multitrain-multimethod matrix. *Psychological Bulletin*, 1959, *56*, 81–105.
Campbell, D. T., & Stanley, J. C. *Experimental and quasi-experimental designs for research.* Chicago: Rand McNally, 1966.
Cannell, C. F., Lawson, S. A., & Hausser, D. L. *A technique for evaluating interviewer performance.* Ann Arbor, MI: Survey Research Center, University of Michigan, 1975.
Cook, T. D., & Campbell, D. T. *Quasi-experimentation: Design and analysis issues for field settings.* Chicago: Rand McNally, 1979.
Cronbach, L. J., & Associates. *Toward reform of program evaluation.* San Francisco: Jossey-Bass, 1980.
Dillman, D. A. *Mail and telephone survey.* New York: Wiley, 1978.
Etzioni, A. Two approaches to organizational analysis: A critique and a suggestion. In H. C. Schulberg, A. Sheldon & F. Baker (Eds.), *Program evaluation in the health fields.* New York: Behavioral Publications, 1969.
Flaherty, E. W., & Morell, J. A. Evaluation: Manifestations of a new field. *Evaluation and Program Planning*, 1978, *1*, 1–10.
Freeman, H. E., & Solomon, M. A. The next decade in evaluation research. *Evaluation and Program Planning*, 1979, *2*, 255–262.
Gruender, D. C. On distinguishing science and technology. *Technology and Culture*, 1971, *12*, 456–463.
Havlock, M. C. *Planning for innovation through the dissemination and utilization of knowledge* (2nd ed.). Ann Arbor, MI: Institute for Social Research, University of Michigan, 1979.
Havlock, R. G., & Havlock, M. C. *Training for change agents.* Ann Arbor, MI: Institute for Social Research, University of Michigan, 1973.
Human Interaction Research Institute. *Putting knowledge to use: A distillation of the literature regarding knowledge transfer and change.* Los Angeles: Human Interaction Research Institute, 1976.
Ingle, M. D., & Klauss, R. Competency based program evaluation: A contingency approach. *Evaluation and Program Planning*, in press.

Kaplan, A. *The conduct of inquiry: Methodology for behavioral science.* Scranton, PA: Chandler, 1964.

Lakatos, I. Falsification and the methodology of scientific research programs. In I. Lakatos & A. Musgrave (Eds.), *Criticism and the growth of knowledge.* London: Cambridge University Press, 1972.

Lucas, H. C., Jr. *Why information systems fail.* New York: Columbia University Press, 1975.

Marcus, A. C. et al. An analytical review of longitudinal and related studies as they apply to the educational process. In *Methodological Foundations for the Study of School Effects* (Vol. 3). Washington, D.C.: National Center for Educational Statistics (DHEW/OE), 1972.

Mischel, W. On the interface of cognition and personality. *American Psychologist,* 1979, *34,* 740–754.

Morell, J. A. The conflict between social research and mental health services. *Administration in Mental Health,* 1977, *4,* 52–58.

Morell, J. A. Followup research as an evaluation strategy. In T. Abramson & C. K. Tittle (Eds.), *Handbook of vocational education evaluation.* Beverly Hills, CA: Sage Publications, 1979. (a)

Morell, J. A. *Program evaluation in social research.* Elmsford, NY: Pergamon Press, 1979. (b)

Moser, C. A., & Kalton, G. *Survey methods in social investigation* (2nd ed.). New York: Basic Books, 1972.

Patton, M. Q. *Utilization focused evaluation.* Beverly Hills, CA: Sage Publications, 1978.

Patton, M. Q. *Qualitative evaluation research.* Beverly Hills, CA: Sage Publications, 1980.

Riecken, H. Memorandum on program evaluation. In C. H. Weiss (Ed.), *Evaluating action programs: Readings in social action research.* Boston: Allyn and Bacon, 1972.

Riecken, H. W., & Boruch, R. F. (Eds.) *Social experimentation: A method for planning and evaluating social intervention.* New York: Academic Press, 1974.

Schatzman, L., & Strauss, A. L. *Field research: Strategies for a natural sociology.* Englewood Cliffs, NJ: Prentice-Hall, 1973.

Selltiz, C., Wrightsman, L. S., & Cook, S. W. *Research methods in social relationsh.* New York: Holt, Rinehart and Winston, Inc., 1976.

Snapper, K. J., & Seaver, D. A. The use of evaluation models for decision making: Application to the community anti-crime program. *Evaluation and Program Planning,* in press.

Strupp, H. H., & Hadley, S. W. A tripartite model of mental health and therapeutic outcomes. *American Psychologist,* 1977, *32,* 187–196.

Suchman, E. A. *Evaluative research.* New York: Russell Sage Foundation, 1967.

Sudman, S. *Applied sampling.* New York: Academic Press, 1976.

Symposium on optimizing, implementing and evaluating public policy. Policy Studies Journal, 1980, special issue 3, 1087–1159.

Thorndike, R. L. *Educational measurement* (2nd ed.). Washington, D.C.: American Council on Education, 1971.

Tripodi, T., Fellin, P., & Epstein, E. *Social program evaluation: Guidelines for health, education and welfare administrators.* Itasca, IL: F. E. Peacock, 1971.

Weiss, C. H. The politicization of evaluation research. In C. H. Weiss (Ed.), *Evaluating action programs: Readings in social action research.* Boston: Allyn and Bacon, 1972.

Weiss, C. H. Knowledge creep and decision accretion. *Knowledge,* 1980, *1,* 381–404.

Wildavsky, A. The self evaluating organization. *Public Administration Review,* 1972, *32,* 509–520.

Williams, W. Implementation analysis and assessment. In W. Williams & R. F. Elmore (Eds.), *Social program implementation*. New York: Academic Press, 1976.
Windle, C., & Neigher, W. Ethical problems in program evaluation: Advice for trapped evaluators. *Evaluation and Program Planning*, 1978, *1*, 97–107.

PREVENTIVE INTERVENTION DURING THE PERINATAL AND INFANCY PERIODS: OVERVIEW AND GUIDELINES FOR EVALUATION

Bernard J. Shuman
Frank Masterpasqua

ABSTRACT. This paper reviews recent changes in perspectives of development in the prenatal, neonatal, and infancy periods and describes exemplary preventive interventions and their evaluation. Particular emphasis is placed on expanding criteria for successful early interventions to include measures of socioemotional and physical health as well as the more traditional measures of intellectual development. A theme which emerges is the need for peer and professional support for early parenting.

For mental health professionals in 1980, it seems natural that the bulk of our attempts at preventive interventions should be focused on the very young. The widespread contemporary assumption "the earlier the better" with regard to intervention stems in large part from the premise that early experience plays an important role in the course of ontogeny. It is important to recall, however, that until fairly recently, children were seen as essentially miniature adults (Aries, 1962) whose development was preformed or predetermined exclusive of the influence of experiential factors (Ausubel, 1970). Only with the writings of Freud (1915) and psychologists such as Hebb (1949) has early experience been viewed as pivotal in shaping development. Indeed, Lorenz's (1965) find-

Bernard J. Shuman, MD is Associate Professor, Department of Mental Health Sciences, Hahnemann Medical College and Hospital; Medical Director, Consultation and Education Services, and Director, Center for the Urban Child, John F. Kennedy Community Mental Health/Mental Retardation Center, 112 North Broad Street, Philadelphia, PA 19102. Frank Masterpasqua, PhD, is Assistant Clinical Professor, Department of Mental Health Sciences, Hahnemann Medical College and Hospital; Assistant Director, Consultation and Education Services, and Associate Director, Center for the Urban Child, John F. Kennedy Community Mental Health/Mental Retardation Center. Reprints may be requested from Bernard J. Shuman, 112 North Broad Street, 7th Floor, Philadelphia, PA 19102.

Prevention in Human Services, Vol. 1(1/2), Fall/Winter 1981

ings that birds can be imprinted to an adult-like figure *only* during a particular period convinced many developmentalists that early experience was not only important, but critical.

There appears to be no final answer to the question of precisely how significant early experience is. Some contemporary writers (e.g., White, 1975) seem convinced that the first 3 years of life do, in fact, represent a critical period in humans. For others (e.g., Kagan, Kearsley, & Zelazo, 1978), the significance of early experience has been overemphasized. It is beyond the scope of this article to discuss the theoretical merits of either stance with regard to early experience. Nonetheless, we believe it important that professionals interested in providing preventive services to the young have some appreciation for the relative reversibility or irreversibility of their efforts.

The most reasonable conclusion to be derived from the literature seems to be that there is little support for the notion of critical periods. "Except for the receptor systems, and most of the evidence concerns the visual system, it is doubtful that truly critical periods exist in human development" (Hunt, 1979, p. 124). Rather, Hunt's review of the early experience literature indicates that there are sensitive periods of human development during which particular events are most influential in establishing patterns of behavior (e.g., the availability of a mother figure during the second 6 months of life). Moreover, "the longer a young organism lives with experience of a given development-fostering quality, the more difficult it is to change the effect" (Hunt, 1979, p. 124).

For preventive interventionists, the implications are twofold. First, we must be attuned to the needs of early sensitive periods so as to provide developmentally responsive environments which help in the establishment of adaptive patterns of behavior. Second, although change becomes more difficult the longer one waits to provide responsive environments, the patterns of behavior which occur partially as a result of early experiences are not irreversible; we are resilient. The view that early development consists of sensitive periods is a theme which will be carried through the present overview.

A second theme which emerges from a review of the more recent literature, and one which may be related to the resilience in development, is the perspective that the newborn is competent in its transactions with the environment (Stone, Smith, & Murphy, 1973). As few as 15 years ago, the widespread assumption concerning early development was that the infant was a "blank slate" ready to be shaped by environmental forces. Beginning with the work of Fantz (1965), Thomas, Chess and Birch (1968), and others, researchers have provided data which demonstrate the often subtle but profound ways in which the young infant plays an active role in its own social and cognitive development. The idea of the infant as competent is a second premise which should be acknowledged in the creation and evaluation of early intervention programs.

General Guidelines for Evaluating Early Intervention

The most widely used means for evaluating the success of early interventions has been the developmental (DQ) or intelligence quotient (IQ). Recently, Zigler and Trickett (1979) criticized the use of the IQ as the sole criterion of such efforts. These authors recommended four parameters of social competence, including IQ, which should be used to assess effectiveness. These are physical health, cognitive development (e.g., DQ, Uzgiris and Hunt's 1975 scale), social/emotional development, (e.g., Ainsworth's, 1978 scale of infant attachment), and measures of achievement (e.g., Caldwell's Cooperative Preschool Inventory, 1970). While it may be impossible for every early prevention effort to address each of these evaluative dimensions, Zigler and Trickett's recommendation for a broadening of the objectives of early preventive programs seems to have merit on at least two grounds. First, conceptually, the parameters more accurately reflect current understanding of the full range of influences on early development. Second, pragmatically, IQ has not been found to be especially useful in predicting such behaviors as social maturity, productivity as a citizen, etc. As a result, funding sources are becoming wary of the DQ/IQ as the sole measure of early interventions.

In the current paper, physical health, cognitive, and social/ emotional development will be used as a basis for describing and evaluating prevention programs during the prenatal, neonatal, and infancy periods.

Prenatal Period: Ensuring a Good Beginning

Obstetrical Care

There is a good deal of evidence which indicates that obstetric care plays an important role in the physical health of the mother and the fetus and in the subsequent development of the child.

Documentation for this conclusion can be found in a recent national perinatal study (Broman, Nichols, and Kennedy, 1975) consisting of over 26,000 children from urban clinics nationwide: 47% were black; 45%, white; and 7%, Puerto Rican. The median SES was 15% below that of the U.S. population of a comparable age. It was found that

> mean I.Q.'s were significantly higher among children of mothers who had more prenatal visits, whose pregnancy was less advanced at time of registration for prenatal care, and who were not anemic during pregnancy. IQ's were also significantly higher among children whose mothers had longer pregnancies (up to 43 weeks), moderate weight gains, no kidney infections, and no hospitalizations during the early part of pregnancy. (p. 245)

While this study used only IQ as the outcome measure, its scope provides evidence for the importance of prenatal care.

Among the poor, for whom prenatal care is most inadequate (Osofsky & Kendall, 1973), the incidence of reproductive risk factors such as prematurity, hypertension, bleeding, etc. are highest, and the relatively high U.S. infant mortality rate is an indictment of our health care priorities. *These statistics call out for programs whose major objective is to reach out to mothers during pregnancy so as to increase their obstetric care.* In one program (Hermalin, Masterpasqua, Shuman, Morrison, Romano, O'Shea, and Gonzalez, Note 1), an attempt was made to reduce perinatal risk factors among young, low-income, inner-city pregnant women through home outreach to ensure adequate obstetric care. Results indicated that 100% of the mothers who received adequate prenatal care, including childbirth education, gave birth to a viable baby within 37–41 weeks of conception. Only 82% of nonparticipants achieved such viability (p. < 006). Also, 100% of the children born to participating mothers attained stable independent respirations within 5 minutes postpartum, while only 70.4% of the other group attained stability within this period (p. < 001).

Traditional measures to evaluate outcome of pregnancy for mother and child have been birth weight, APGAR score, and gestational age. While each of these measures has merit, a more comprehensive profile of pregnancy, labor, and delivery outcome can be attained from Littman and Parmelee's (Note 2) Obstetric Complication Scale (OCS) and Postnatal Complication Scale (PCS). The OCS consists of 41 items obtainable from the mother's prenatal and labor and delivery records and yields a standardized score ranging from 50 to 160. Field, Hallock, Ting, Dempsey, Dabiri and Shuman (1978) found that OCS and PCS were among the most efficient and accurate predictors of continuing psychological risk beyond the neonatal period.

Childbirth Education

Since the beginnings of natural childbirth education (Lamaze method) in Britain and the Soviet Union in the 1930s, preparation for childbirth has become a widespread practice in the United States. The original objective of natural childbirth was to reduce birth pain without the use of anesthesia through didactic instruction in the anatomy and physiology of the birth process and through training for breathing and relaxation during labor.

Subsequently, based on the assumption that medication given to nonprepared women has a negative impact on fetuses, a number of researchers have attempted to demonstrate that preparation for childbirth reduces reproductive risk. Beck and Hall (1978) identified five major problem areas in the design of these studies which render conclusions concerning the medical outcome of prepared childbirth tenuous. First, many of the findings were anecdotally recorded without the use of control groups. Second, the problem of subject self-selection (i.e., the possibility that outcome is attributable to motivational differences between selectees and nonselectees) was common. The third problem cited by Beck and Hall was the absence of an attention placebo control group in any of the evaluations. Fourth, it has seldom been explicated as to whether obstetricians and/or observers were aware of the type of prenatal preparation mothers received. Therefore, results may be attributable to observer bias. Fifth, in many studies statistical analyses and detailed procedures were lacking, making it difficult to precisely replicate or validate findings.

Despite these methodological limitations, Beck and Hall found that, particularly among recent studies, there has been no consistent trend to indicate medical benefits attributable to childbirth education. Failure to find medical effects may be due to the recent routine reduction in the use of obstetrical medication in recent years, even for women not enrolled in childbirth education classes. Therefore, the original notion that natural childbirth might reduce reproductive risk by decreasing harmful effects of medication is no longer as tenable.

In spite of the absence of findings of medical benefits due to preparation for childbirth, there is reason to believe that the support and information given to mothers prior to delivery may have a subsequent psychological impact.

> Far more subtle benefits of the [childbirth] training program may be found if mothers' and fathers' relationships and treatment for their newborns were assessed. The ability of the mother to be awake during delivery and to greet offspring at the point of birth has been given measured importance in establishing a healthy child-rearing environment. (Zax, Sameroff, & Farnum, 1975, p. 190)

The "measured importance" to which Zax et al. refer is reflected in the work of Klaus and Kennell (1976) who found that early mother-newborn contact is important in the establishment of a healthy child-rearing environment.

A recent study by one of the authors (Masterpasqua, Note 3) showed that, as assessed by Broussard and Hartner's Neonatal Perception Inventory (1970), mothers who received childbirth education had enhanced perceptions of their newborns (i.e., there were fewer mothers in the prepared groups who believed they would have more difficulties with their own infants as compared with the average baby). Since, in that study, prepared mothers were no less medicated than nonprepared mothers, reduction in the use of medication can not be used to explain these results. Further studies are required to determine how the knowledge acquired during childbirth education affects maternal perceptions during the neonatal period.

Pregnancy and the birth of the child are potentially stressful life events for all parents; for the many young parents in our society without family and neighborhood supports, these experiences can be especially troublesome. A number of authors have emphasized the importance of social supports during such "normative developmental crises," or major life changes (e.g., Caplan, 1974; Hirsch, 1980). "Chief among the factors hypothesized to moderate the relationship between life change and symptom development has been the presence of helpful natural support systems" (Hirsch, 1980, p. 50). Preparedness for childbirth may not only serve to provide anticipatory guidance for expectant parents, but may also be an avenue for the creation of peer and professional support systems during a sensitive period in parent-child relationships. The support thus provided may enhance mothers' sense of confidence in being able to cope with a new baby.

Our discussion of childbirth education implies two guidelines for implementation and evaluation of early intervention. First, in addition to the focus on the physical aspects of the birth process, childbirth education classes should more directly address the psychological aspects of pregnancy and the birth process. Second, in evaluating these programs, outcome measures should include assessments of the psychological aspects of the birth process. Two such assessment measures are the Maternal Attitude to Pregnancy Inventory (Blau, Wilkowitz, & Cohen, 1964), which can provide a baseline for assessing the mother's initial perceptions and feelings about the pregnancy, and the Neonatal Perception Inventory (Broussard & Hartner, 1970), which can help determine the impact of the intervention.

Neonatal Period

In our discussion of the prenatal period, emphasis was placed on the need to reduce reproductive risk factors and the potential impact of such factors upon subsequent development. Nonetheless, it is important to recall the contemporary notion that the effects of early experiential factors, such as reproductive risk, are not irrevocable. Sameroff and Chandler (1975), in their review of the long-term effects of reproductive risks, concluded that the effects of early perinatal complications can be exacerbated or ameliorated depending upon the subsequent caretaking environment. For example, the long-term effects of an early risk factor such as prematurity may in some measure depend upon the parents' attitudes and responses toward their premature baby. The neonatal period, then, provides the opportunity to lay a foundation for a healthy parent-child relationship and to promote appropriate parental expectations and responsivity to the individual characteristics and needs of the newborn.

The recent increase in interest in the neonatal period can be attributed to at least two lines of influence. The first relates to the notion that even the newborn actively participates in shaping its own social development (Stone, et al., 1973). The second influence is based upon the work of ethologists who have demonstrated the importance of maternal-neonate contact in a variety of mammalian species (Lorenz, 1965). Indeed, this latter aspect appears to have led directly to studies of Ringler, Trause, Klaus, and Kennell (1978) whose recent work indicates "that when most new mothers are with their newborns soon after birth, their infants capture their interest and attention in a way that may not occur when their first encounter begins later" (p. 864). These authors report that extra postpartum contact seems to influence measures of mother-child interaction as much as 5 years after birth. These studies have provided a scientific basis for early mother-neonate contact and have stimulated changes in hospital postpartum procedures to accommodate this need.

In addition to studies of the importance of contact between mother and newborn, a great deal of emphasis has been placed upon study of individual characteristics of neonates and how such attributes influence the interaction between parent and infant. Chief among the measures of early individual difference has been the Brazelton (1973) Neonatal Behavior Assessment Scale (NBAS).

> The examination procedure encompasses an attempt to re-capitulate experiences which will be typical of future interac-tive situations. Normal newborns are manipulated in such a way that over the course of the half hour examination they exhibit motor, cognitive, social and temperamental responses as well as observable psychophysiological reactions. These are elicited, observed and measured by the examiner in a way that might represent or duplicate the responses of a caring mother and father. Thus, the scoring becomes a way of assessing the capacity for interaction on the part of the baby which might be expected by his or her environment. The response of an examiner to the particular infant then be-comes a measure of prediction of the environment's response to the same infant. (Brazelton, 1978, p. 3)

A wide range of factors have been shown to influence the Brazelton score of performance. For example, Aleksandrowicz & Aleksandrowicz (1974) reported close relationships between ob-stetric medication and items on Brazelton's NBAS such as habitu-ation, cuddliness, and smiles. Strauss, Lessen-Firestone, Starr, and Ostrea (1975) found narcotics-addicted newborns to be deficient in learning and orienting. In turn, Osofsky and Danzger (1974) reported that infants' NBAS scores were related to patterns of mother-newborn interaction.

These recent findings concerning early individual behavioral differences point to the need for intervention to alert parents to the characteristics of their newborns and to provide some options in caretaking which accommodate the behavioral idiosyncracies of babies. Toward this goal, Field, Dempsey, Hallock, and Shuman

(1978) recently adapted the Brazelton Scale into a mother's assessment of the behavior of her infant (MABI) which closely correlates with the NBAS and appears useful in preparing mothers for the unique attributes of their neonates.

Neonatal behavioral evaluations have also been used to predict abnormal parenting practices. Gray, Cutler, Dean, and Kempe (1976) used four screening procedures at discrete intervals to determine the correlation between the neonatal caretaking environment and subsequent parenting practices. These were: (1) collection of prenatal information (e.g., feelings about the pregnancy, expectations for the newborn child); (2) administration of a questionnaire during a prenatal or early postnatal period (these questions were similar to those obtained in the prenatal interview); (3) assessment of labor and delivery room information in which the first encounter between mother and infant was observed and recorded, including videotaping of the mother and infant interaction and any other anecdotal information from the delivery room staff; and (4) observation and/or interview during the postpartum period (to obtain or expand on information gained during the prenatal period). From these data, groups were broken down into high-risk with intervention, high-risk nonintervention, and low-risk control groups.

When the children were a mean age of 26.8 months, a home visit was made to 25 families selected at random in each of these categories. At this time, abnormal parenting practices were defined using various measures of child abuse, neglect, and the child's performance on the Denver Developmental Screening test. Among the 50 home-visited in the two high-risk groups, there were 22 indications of abnormal parenting practices and only 2 indications in the control group of 25 (p < .01). Moreover, comprehensive pediatric care by the same physician, visits on a weekly basis by a home visitor, and frequent telephone contact between the physician and family provided to the high-risk intervention group prevented, to a significant degree, abnormal parenting practices.

Implications of this study are twofold. First, information gained from observations in the labor and delivery room was the best predictor of subsequent abnormal parenting practices, while the questionnaires did not add significantly to the accuracy of prediction. Gray et al. (1976) recognized that delivery room observations may not be feasible, but noted that evaluation during "the early post-partum period affords the best opportunity for collection and analysis of prenatal, labor and delivery and post-partum observations. Such observations are non-invasive and should be part of the obstetrical and postpartum routine" (p. 9).

Infancy Period

The contemporary perspective regarding infancy is that the initial 12 to 18 months consist of dynamic interplay of two behavioral systems: attachment and the need for exploration/separation (e.g., Ainsworth, Blehar, Waters, & Wall, 1978; Mahler, Pine, & Bergman, 1975). The infant comes into the world equipped with a behavioral repertoire which appears to ensure that attachment will occur. These behaviors include crying, grasping, looking, smiling, sucking, etc. (Bowlby, 1969). It follows that the major task for parents in the formation of an early, secure, strong attachment is responsivity to these behaviors. More importantly, this responsivity should be synchronized with the particular behavioral rhythms and characteristics of the infant.

For instance, a study by Bell and Ainsworth (1972) indicates how behavioral responsivity can lead to more effective patterns of parenting and attachment. These authors found that when mothers responded quickly and consistently to their infants' cries during the first 3 months of life, these babies were less likely to cry during the last 3 months of the first year and tended to be more communicative at 1 year than babies whose mothers did not respond to the cries consistently or rapidly. In another study, Blehar, Lieberman, and Ainsworth (1977) found that infants later identified as securely attached (see Ainsworth, et al., 1978) were more responsive in early en face encounters than infants judged to be anxiously attached, and their mothers were more contingently responsive and encouraging of interaction. Infants later identified as anxiously attached were more unresponsive and negative in early en face interactions than securely attached infants, and their mothers were more likely to be impassive or abrupt, i.e., lacking in synchrony.

Early Intervention Programs for the Promotion of DQ/IQ

The value of assessing early parent-infant mutual responsivity/synchrony has only recently been recognized. Programs have been almost exclusively devoted to evaluating the impact of early stimulation or intervention upon IQ or DQ, and a number of excellent reviews are available which describe the impact of these efforts (Bronfenbrenner, 1975; Horowitz & Paden, 1973). These reviews suggest that early intervention can be effective if a number of criteria are met: (1) intervention should begin at the earliest possible time—prenatally, if possible; (2) "priority, status and support" (Bronfenbrenner, 1975) should be given to the mother/ child system; (3) parents should be actively involved as the primary teachers of their children; and (4) intervention should be ecological in nature (i.e., should be responsive to real life needs of low-income parents, including health care, housing, etc.). Reference is made to Heber, Garber, Harrington, and Hoffman (Note 4), Levenstein (Note 5), and Gordon (Note 6) as representative of programs which have met some or all of these criteria and have had substantial impact on early intellectual development.

Recently Developed Measures of Socioemotional Development

As recommended at the outset of the paper, programs in early intervention need to address socioemotional as well as intellectual development. To this end, a number of instruments have been developed in recent years to evaluate patterns of parent-infant synchrony and mutual responsivity. In addition to serving as a means for evaluation, these instruments can be effectively used to provide baseline and follow-up information for preventive interventions. For the most part, these assessment measures have focused on two aspects of early socioemotional development: (1) innate individual behavioral and temperamental differences which play a role in parent-infant interaction (see Brazelton, 1973; Thomas, Chess, & Birch, 1968) and (2) direct observations of mother-infant interaction (e.g., Ainsworth, 1973).

Carey (1970) developed a method for measuring infant tempera-ment which can be helpful in alerting parents to particular tem-peramental characteristics of their babies. The instrument con-sists of questions asked of parents around nine dimensions of temperament (e.g., activity, threshold, intensity, distractibility). Ainsworth (1973) developed a scale which can be used beginning in the first few months of life to assess behavior and interactions such as mother's synchronization of feeding to baby's pace, appropriate-ness of mother's initiations of interactions, mother's delight in baby, etc. Maisie and Campbell (Note 7) created an instrument which can be used by physicians, nurses, and other health practi-tioners during pediatric examinations to assess the quality of attachment between mother and infant.

Early Intervention Programs for the Promotion of Socioemotional
Development

Two recent programs appear to have recognized the significance
of evaluating the socioemotional as well as cognitive results of
early preventive interventions Field, Widmayer, Springer, and
Ignatoff, (1980) reported on a program for the preterm infants of
lower SES black mothers. Teenage mothers provided with home-
based infant enrichment activities were compared with controls of
term infants of teenage mothers and of preterm infants of older
mothers. Mothers who received intervention had infants who
showed enhanced scores on measures of infant temperament, face-
to-face interaction with their mothers at 4 months, as well as on
Denver scores. In addition, at 4 months treatment, mothers had
more realistic expectations of developmental milestones and child-
rearing attitudes, and at 8 months, the intervention group had
superior Bayley and infant temperament scores. In a second study,
Bromwich and Parmelee (1979) found that home visits increased
parental responsiveness to their preterm infants and enhanced
home observation measures (Beckwith, Note 8) of mother-infant
interaction at 24 months. In addition to demonstrating the effects
of early intervention on socioemotional development, both studies
exemplify the importance of support for the parenting role through
regular home visits.

Measuring the Quality of Attachment at 1 Year and its
Relationship to Ego-Resilience

Toward the end of the first year, the infant's ability to independently explore his/her social and physical environment while using
the mother as a home base takes on considerable significance. We
have already noted that the quality of this attachment has been
found to be related to the kind of parenting activities experienced
early in the first year (e.g., Bell and Ainsworth, 1972). A number of
more recent studies indicate further that the relative security of
the attachment at around 12–18 months is predictive of the social
competence and ego-resilience at the preschool age.

Ainsworth, Blehar, Waters, and Wall (1978) have developed a
system to measure the quality of the baby's attachment in terms of
its balance with his/her need to explore. The Ainsworth et al.
system identifies three major patterns of attachment: securely
attached infants; anxiously attached, avoidant infants; and anxi-

ously attached, ambivalent infants. Only the first group shows good adaptation. In a recent series of studies using the Ainsworth et al. scale, Arend, Gove, and Sroufe (1979) have demonstrated that infants with a secure attachment are more likely to show enhanced social problem-solving abilities and have increased scores of measures of ego-resilience and ego-control as preschoolers. In another study demonstrating the relationship between social supports, stressful life events, and parenting, Vaughn, Egland, Sroufe, and Waters (1979) found "anxious attachment is associated with less stable caretaking environments than secure attachment; change from secure to anxious attachment was associated with higher stressful events scores than stable secure attachment" (p. 971).

Based on the work of Ainsworth, Sroufe, and their colleagues, two recommendations for intervention can be derived. First, programs need to be created which use quality of attachment at 12 and 18 months as criteria for successful intervention. Second, an important ingredient in ensuring quality attachment is likely to be the provision of support to parents in order to stabilize the caretaking environment.

Summary and Conclusions

In this brief overview of recent perspectives on early development, intervention, and evaluation, emphasis has been placed on a few key concepts. First, early development appears to consist of sensitive, rather than critical, periods. Second, early behavior seems to emerge from a transaction between an inherently active, young individual and his/her social and physical world. Third, means of evaluation need to be expanded to include physical and socioemotional as well as intellectual development. These concepts have been reflected in discussions of interventions and evaluations during prenatal, neonatal, and infant development. During the prenatal period, the importance of outreach to ensure adequate medical care was posited, and it was suggested that programs designed to meet this need be evaluated through the use of Littman and Parmelee's Obstetric Complication Scale (OCS) and Postnatal Complications Scale (PCS). In addition, emphasis was placed upon the importance of prepared childbirth and its potential impact on mothers' feelings about being able to cope with their newborns. There are a number of scales which can be used to assess the early relationship (e.g., the Neonatal Perception Inventory and the Maternal Attitudes Toward Pregnancy Inventory).

The discussion of the neonatal period focused on three major preventive and evaluative issues. First, the accommodation of hospital procedures to allow for early mother-newborn contact is needed. Second, it is important to support new parents by providing them with information concerning the unique attributes of their infants and by suggesting ways in which parents might best respond to those characteristics. One important means of identifying individual differences in behavior at birth has been Brazelton's Neonatal Behavior Assessment Scale which has been found to relate to a number of early influences as well as patterns of mother-newborn interaction. A third issue concerned the use of screening instruments during the neonatal period to detect abnormal parenting patterns. Toward this end, the work of Gray et al.(1979) provides a tool which can be used in maternity pavillions for mothers who may be in need of intervention and support.

In the section on infant interventions, particular emphasis was placed on programs and evaluations which address the full range of infant behavior, including intellectual and socioemotional development. There is considerable evidence to suggest that programs which support the parenting role can be especially effective when measured by instruments such as Ainsworth's Scale of parent-infant interaction. Moreover, there is now empirical support for the notion that the quality of this parent-infant attachment at 12 months relates to subsequent preschool-age characteristics such as ego-resilience and interpersonal problem solving abilities.

REFERENCE NOTES

1.   Hermalin, J., Masterpasqua, F., Shuman, B. J., Morrison, I., Romano, M., O'Shea, L., & Gonzalez, R. *Reducing the complications of labor and delivery: The effectiveness of the Lamaze technique for Hispanic mothers.* Manuscript submitted for publication, 1980.
2.   Littman, B., & Parmelee, A. *The obstetric complications scales and postnatal complications scales.* Unpublished manuscript, 1974. (Available from Department of Pediatrics, Division of Child Development, School of Medicine, University of California. Los Angeles, CA, 90024).
3.   Masterpasqua, F. *The effectiveness of prepared childbirth as an early intervention technique.* Unpublished doctoral dissertation, Rutgers University, 1980.
4.   Heber, R., Garber, H., Harrington, S., & Hoffman, C. *Rehabilitation of families at risk for mental retardation.* Madison, WI: University of Wisconsin, Rehabilitation Research and Training Center in Mental Retardation, December 1972.
5.   Levenstein, P. *Verbal interaction project.* Mineola, NY: Family Service Association of Nassau County, Inc. 1972.
6.   Gordon, I. J. *A home learning center approach to early stimulation.* Gainesville, FL: University of Florida, Institute for Development of Human Resources, 1972.

7.   Maisie, H. N., & Campbell, B. K. *The attachment indicators during stress scale*. San Francisco: Childrens Hospital & Medical Center of San Francisco, CA, 1977.
8.   Beckwith, L. Receptive language in preterm infants: Antecedents and correlates in caregiver interaction. In *Precursors and correlates of two-year-old competence in preterm infants*. Symposium presented at the meeting of Society for Research in Child Development, New Orleans, March 1977.

REFERENCES

Ainsworth, M. D. S. System for rating maternal care behavior. In E. Gil Boyer (Ed.), *Measures of maturation* (Vol. 1). Philadelphia: Humanizing Learning Program for Better Schools, Inc., 1973.
Ainsworth, M. D. S., Blehar, M. C., Waters, E., & Wall, S. *Patterns of attachment: A psychological study of the strange situation*. Hillsdale, NJ: Lawrence Erlbaum, 1978.
Aleksandrowicz, M. K., & Aleksandrowicz, D. R. Obstetrical pain-relieving drugs as predictors of infant behavior variability. *Child Development*, 1974, *45*, 935–45.
Arend, R., Gove, F. L., & Sroufe, L. A. Continuity of individual adaptation from infancy to kindergarten: A predictive study of ego-resiliency and curiosity in preschoolers. *Child Development*, 1979, *50*, 950–959.
Aries, P. *Centuries of childhood*. New York: Knopf, 1962.
Ausubel, D. P., & Sullivan, E. V. *Theory and problems of child development*. New York: Grune & Stratton, 1970.
Beck, N. C., & Hall, D. Natural childbirth: A review and analysis. *Obstetrics and Gynecology*, 1978, *52*, 371–379.
Bell, S., & Ainsworth, M. D. S. Infant crying and maternal responsiveness. *Child Development*, 1972, *43*, 1171–1190.
Blau, A., Wilkowitz, J., & Cohen, J. Maternal attitude to pregnancy instrument: A research test for psychogenic obstetrical complications. A preliminary report. *American Journal of Orthopsychiatry*, 1964, *10*, 324–331.
Blehar, M. C., Lieberman, A. F., & Ainsworth, M. D. S. Early face-to-face interaction and its relation to later infant-mother attachment. *Child Development*, 1977, *48*, 182–194.
Bowlby, J. Attachment. In *Attachment and Loss* (Vol. 1). New York: Basic Books, 1969.
Brazelton, T. B. Neonatal behavioral assessment scale. *Clinics in Developmental Medicine*, No. 50. Philadelphia: Lippincott, 1973.
Brazelton, T. B. A commentary on the Brazelton neonatal behavior assessment scale. In A. J. Sameroff (Ed.), Organization and stability of newborn behavior. *Monographs of the Society for Research in Child Development*, 1978, *43* (5–6, Serial No. 177).
Broman, S. H., Nichols, P. L., & Kennedy, W. A. *Preschool IQ: Prenatal and early developmental correlates*. Hillside, NJ: Lawrence Erlbaum Assoc., 1975.
Bromwich, R. M., & Parmelee, A. H. An intervention program for pre-term infants. In T. M. Field (Ed.), *Infants born at risk: Behavior and development*. New York: SP Medical and Scientific Books, 1979.
Bronfenbrenner, U. Is early intervention effective? In B. Friedlander, G. M. Sterritt, & G. E. Kirk (Eds.). *Exceptional infant: Assessment & intervention* (Vol. 3). New York: Brunner/Mazel, 1975.
Broussard, E. R., & Hartner, M. S. S. Maternal perception of the neonate as related to development. *Child Psychiatry and Human Development*, 1970, *1*, 16–25.
Caldwell, B. M. *Cooperative preschool inventory*. (Rev. Ed.). Menlo Park, CA: Addison-Wesley Publishing Co., 1970.

Caplan, G. *Social systems and community mental health*. New York: Behavioral Publications, 1974.

Carey, W. B. A simplified method for measuring infant temperament. *Journal of Pediatrics*, 1970, *77*, 188–194.

Fantz, R. L. Visual perception from birth as shown by pattern selectivity. *Annals of the New York Academy of Sciences*, 1965, *118*, 793–814.

Field, T. M., Dempsey, J. R., Hallock, N. H., & Shuman, H. H. The mother's assessment of the behavior of her infant. *Infant Behavior & Development*, 1978, *1*, 156–167.

Field, T., Hallock, N., Ting, G., Dempsey, J., Dabiri, C., & Shuman, H. H. A first-year follow-up of high-risk infants: Formulating a cumulative risk index. *Child Development*, 1978, *49*, 119–131.

Field, T. M., Widmayer, S. M., Springer, S., & Ignatoff, E. Teenage, lower-class, black mothers and their pre-term infants: An intervention and developmental follow-up. *Child Development*, 1980, *51*, 426–436.

Freud, S. *Instincts and their vicissitudes*. In *Collected Papers*, 1915, *4*, 60–83. London: Hogarth, 1950.

Gray, J. D., Cutler, C. A., Dean, J. G., & Kempe, C. H. Prediction and prevention of child abuse and neglect. *Journal of Social Issues*, 1979, *35*, 127–139.

Hebb, D. O. *The organization of behavior*. New York: Wiley 1949.

Hirsch, B. J. Natural support systems and coping with major life changes. *American Journal of Community Psychology*, 1980, *8*, 159–172.

Horowitz, F. D., & Paden, L. Y. The effectiveness of environmental intervention programs. In B. M. Caldwell & H. N. Ricciuti (Eds.), *Review of Child Development Research* (Vol. 3). Chicago: University of Chicago Press, 1973.

Hunt, J. M. Psychological development: Early experience. In M. R. Rosenzweig & L. W. Porter (Eds.), *Annual Review of Psychology*, 1979, *30*.

Kagan, J., Kearsley, R. B., & Zelazo, P. R. *Infancy: Its place in human development*. Cambridge, MA: Harvard University Press, 1978.

Klaus, M. H., & Kennell, J. H. *Maternal infant bonding*. St. Louis, MO: C. V. Mosby, 1976.

Lorenz, K. *Evolution and modification of behavior*. Chicago: University of Chicago Press, 1965.

Mahler, M. S., Pine, F., & Bergman, A. *The psychological birth of the human infant*. New York: Basic Books, 1975.

Osofsky, H. S., & Kendall, N. Poverty as a criterion of risk. *Clinical Obstetrics and Gynecology*, 1973, *10*, 103–119.

Osofsky, J. D., & Danzger, B. Relationships between neonatal characteristics and mother-infant interaction. *Developmental Psychology*, 1974, *10*, 124–130.

Ringler, N., Trause, M. A., Klaus, M., & Kennell, J. The effects of extra post-partum contact and maternal speech patterns on children's IQ's, speech, and language comprehension at five. *Child Development*, 1978, *49*, 862–865.

Sameroff, A. J., & Chandler, M. J. Reproductive risk and the continuum of caretaking casualty. In F. D. Horowitz, M. Hetherington, S. Scarr-Salapatek, & G. Siegel (Eds.), *Review of Child Development Research*. Chicago: University of Chicago Press, 1975.

Stone, L. J., Smith, H. T., & Murphy, L. B. *The competent infant: Research and commentary*. New York: Basic Books, 1973.

Strauss, M. E., Lessen-Firestone, J. K., Starr, R. H., & Ostrea, E. M. Behavior of narcotics addicted newborns. *Child Development*, 1975, *46*, 887–893.

Thomas, A., Chess, S., & Birch, H. G. *Temperament and behavior disorders in children*. New York: New York University Press, 1968.

Uzgiris, I. C., & Hunt, J. McV. *Assessment in infancy: Ordinal scales of psychological development*. Chicago: University of Illinois Press, 1975.

Vaughn, B., Edgland, B., Sroufe, L. A., & Waters, E. Individual differences in infant-mother attachment at 12 and 18 months: Stability and change in families under stress. *Child Development*, 1979, *50*, 971–975.

White, B. L. *The first three years of life.* Englewood Cliffs, NJ: Prentice-Hall, 1975.

Zax, M., Sameroff, A. J., & Farnum, J. E. Childbirth education: Maternal attitudes and delivery. *American Journal of Obstetrics and Gynecology*, 1975, *123*, 185–190.

Zigler, E., & Trickett, P. K. The role of national policy in promoting social competence in children. In M. W. Whalen & J. E. Rolf (Eds.), *Primary prevention of psychopathology* (Vol. 3). Hanover, NH: University Press of New England, 1979.

FEDERAL REGULATIONS AND THE LIVES OF CHILDREN IN DAY CARE

Jeffrey R. Travers

ABSTRACT. The National Day Care Study investigated relationships between regulatable characteristics of day care centers—in particular, staff/child ratios, group size, and staff qualifications—and the costs and quality of care experienced by preschool children, especially children from low-income families in federally subsidized care. The study found that group size, the total number of children in a classroom, was associated with several measures of the quality of the social environment and of children's development. In small groups, as opposed to large, children were more cooperative, more likely to engage in spontaneous verbalization and creative/intellectual activities, and less likely to wander aimlessly or be uninvolved in activities. They also made more rapid gains on standardized tests of cognitive and linguistic growth. The study further found that caregivers with education or training specifically related to young children showed a relatively high degree of social interaction with children (praising, comforting, responding, questioning, and instructing) and that children in their care made relatively rapid gains on standardized tests. Staff/child ratios were related to some aspects of caregiver behavior, but these relationships were less consistently indicative of quality than those exhibited by group size or caregiver education/training. Because the latter characteristics are relatively low-cost components of day care, the study concluded that the federal government could buy better care at lower cost by giving them greater emphasis in its purchasing standards.

The federal government has become a major purchaser of day care for the children of the working poor. In fiscal 1977, federal expenditures on child care and related services reached almost

---

This paper is based on and partially excerpted from the final report of the National Day Care Study, particularly its first volume, *Children at the Center* (Ruopp, Travers, Glantz, & Coelen, 1979), and its second volume, *Research Results of the National Day Care Study* (Travers, Goodson, Singer, & Connell, 1980), both published by Abt Books, Cambridge, MA. The study was funded by the Administration for Children, Youth and Families, U.S. Department of Health, Education and Welfare and was conducted by Abt Associates, Inc., with SRI International. Allen N. Smith was the Government Project Officer, and Richard R. Ruopp served as Project Director. Reprints may be obtained from Jeffrey R. Travers, Abt Associates, Inc., 55 Wheeler Street, Cambridge, MA 02138.

$2.8 billion and affected over a million children (Congressional Budget Office, 1978).

With the government's increasing financial role has come a concomitant increase in concern about the quality of care purchased with federal dollars, particularly with the developmental effects of subsidized out-of-home care. In part, this concern has been motivated by well-known facts that children from low-income families suffer educational disadvantages relative to their middle-class peers and are at greater risk of illness, delinquency, and other social problems. Advocates have hoped and urged that high-quality child care, providing a range of developmental services, might act as a form of preventive intervention, offsetting some of the risks associated with poverty. While some commentators continue to voice fears that day care per se may be harmful relative to home rearing (e.g., Fraiberg, 1977), the overwhelming weight of contemporary research evidence is that good day care is not harmful and is in some ways beneficial, expecially with respect to school-related cognitive skills in low-income children (Belsky & Steinberg, 1978; Etaugh, 1980). However, the determinants of quality in child care have not been investigated extensively.

Widespread concern over the quality of federally subsidized care gave rise, in 1968, to the Federal Interagency Day Care Requirements (FIDCR), purchasing standards designed to prevent harm and to promote development by setting a floor under the quality of care that could legally be bought with federal dollars. Based largely on expert opinion, the FIDCR cover a variety of characteristics of day care centers and family day care homes, including staff/child ratios, group sizes, staff qualifications, suitability and safety of physical facilities, supplementary services such as health care, and, for centers, formal involvement of parents in policy making, among others. Subsequently, a modified version of the FIDCR was attached to Title XX of the Social Security Act, the single largest funding vehicle for subsidized care, with severe financial penalties to be levied for noncompliance.

Because the FIDCR are more stringent than the licensing codes of most states, particularly in their staff/child ratio requirements,[1] the federal regulations have been attacked as excessively costly. Consequently, in 1974, the Federal Office of Child Development (now the Administration for Children, Youth and Families) funded a large-scale study of the costs and effects associated with variations in regulated characteristics of day care facilities. That investigation, the National Day Care Study (NDCS) was completed in 1978, and in 1979, a summary report of its findings was published (Ruopp, Travers, Glantz, & Coelen, 1979). The report had a clear and direct influence on the revision of the federal day care regulations proposed by the Department of Health, Education and Welfare shortly thereafter (Federal Register, 1980). This article summarizes selected portions of the report, namely, those dealing with relationships between certain regulated characteristics of day care centers serving preschool children and the social experiences and development of those children.

Overview of the National Day Care Study

The NDCS focused on the largest group of children receiving federally subsidized care, children aged 3–5, and on the day care settings in which most of these children are found, urban day care centers serving low-income families. The primary objective of the study was to determine how variations in staff/child ratio, group size, and staff qualifications affect the daily experiences and consequent development of these children as well as the costs of care. These independent variables were highlighted because of their policy importance and presumed likelihood of affecting children. (Other regulatable center characteristics were studied less intensively and will not be discussed here.)

The main cost/effects component of the study, which addressed these issues directly, is described in the section below on design and methods. However, it is important to note that the cost/effects study was part of a larger effort that also included two substudies designed to provide useful supplementary information on characteristics of day care centers nationally and on center care for infants and toddlers. In addition, the research design and methods described here were developed during two preparatory phases which will not be described in detail, but which were essential to the success of the project.

The first of the two supporting studies, the National Day Care Center Supply Study (Coelen, Glantz, & Calore, 1978), was a national telephone survey designed to collect information about enrollment, staffing, costs, and other characteristics of centers. Unlike the cost/effects study, the supply study was limited to those centers primarily serving preschool children. Results were based on a national probability sample of over 3,100 centers, stratified by state. The data provided a profile of center-based care available nationally and by state, as well as estimates of compliance with state and federal regulations. Supply study data also played an important role in projecting the national implications of the results of the cost/effects component of the NDCS and the potential impact of alternative regulations, funding policies, and monitoring practices.

The second supporting study of the NDCS focused on center care arrangements for children under 3. The Infant/Toddler Day Care Study was initiated after the Title XX FIDCR imposed staff/child ratio requirements for centers receiving federal funds to care for infants and toddlers. (The 1968 FIDCR had not established ratio standards for infant-toddler care.) This research effort was designed to provide policymakers with three kinds of data not previously available. First, centers caring for infants and toddlers were surveyed nationally to provide data about their distribution and characteristics, e.g., equipment, staff/child ratios, group sizes, program schedules, and activities. Second, on-site interviews were conducted with selected center directors, caregivers, and parents to gather more detailed data on these center characteristics, as well as opinions about infant and toddler care. Third, selected staff were observed as they cared for infants and toddlers in order to develop a profile of caregiver behavior. Caregiver behavior was examined in relation to staff/child ratio, group size, and caregiver qualifications (Ruopp, et al., 1979, Appendix B).

The NDCS Cost/Effects Study was conducted in three phases. Phase I (July 1974 to September 1975) was devoted to refinement of the study design, to selection of sites and centers, and to initial selection and field testing of study instruments. Atlanta, Detroit, and Seattle were chosen as the study sites, and a total of 64 centers were subsequently selected for participation in Phase II. Phase II (September 1975 to September 1976) was a year-long study of naturally existing relationships between regulatable center characteristics and outcomes for children. The 64 centers were selected for high or low values of staff/child ratio, group size, and staff education. Measures of classroom process, based on observations of caregivers and children, and measures of developmental change, based on standardized tests and rating scales, were administrated in all 64 centers. Data were analyzed to (1) formulate initial hypotheses about relationships among regulatable center characteristics, classroom process, and developmental outcomes and (2) refine the measures of regulatable characteristics, classroom process, and developmental outcomes to be used in Phase III.

Phase III (October 1976 to September 1977) was designed to

address the study's main objective. The Phase III investigation had two components: a 49-center quasi-experiment conducted in all three sites and a randomized experiment conducted in 8 centers operated by the Atlanta Public Schools (APS). (The 8 APS centers were not included in the 49-center sample.) In both studies, selected center characteristics were altered systematically, permitting measurement of the costs and effects associated with such changes.

Design and Methods

Phase III Design

The quasi-experiment was a comparison of three groups of centers (Figure 1). Group I (the "treatment" group) consisted of 14 centers that had low observed staff/child ratios (1:9.1) in Phase II and whose ratios were increased to 1:5.9 in Phase III.[2] Effects of this treatment on caregivers and children were compared with results from a matched group of 14 untreated, low-ratio (1:9.1) centers (Group II) and with those from a group of 21 untreated, high-ratio (1:5.9) centers (Group III). The three sets of ratios applied to classrooms that served primarily 3- and 4-year-old children. In some centers, 3-year-olds were clearly separate from 4-year-olds; in others, the two ages were mixed in the same classroom. No attempt was made in the quasi-experiment to alter natural variations in age grouping. Group size, caregiver experience, and years of education were distributed as evenly as possible across the three experimental groups, so that the effect of ratio could be singled out. Ratio was chosen for manipulation because of its critical policy relevance; manipulation would reduce any confounding between ratio and other center characteristics, permitting relatively clearcut assessment of its effects.

Group I	—	Treated centers
	—	(Observed mean ratio for 14 centers = 1:9.1 in Phase II; ratio raised to 1:5.9 in Phase III)
Group II	—	Untreated low-ratio centers
	—	(Observed mean ratio for 14 centers = 1:9.1)
Group III	—	Untreated high-ratio centers
	—	(Observed mean ratio for 21 centers = 1:5.9)

FIGURE 1.   Design of the 49-center quasi-experiment.

	High Ratio (Observed Mean Ratio = 1:5.4)	Low Ratio (Observed Mean Ratio = 1:7.4)
High Staff Education	4 Classrooms	4 Classrooms
Medium Staff Education	7 Classrooms	4 Classrooms
Low Staff Education	6 Classrooms	4 Classrooms

High staff education: lead teacher was a center director, usually with a master's degree

Medium staff education: lead teacher was a graduate of Atlanta Area Technical School's two-year day care program

Low staff education: lead teacher had not completed the Atlanta Area Technical School's two-year day care program

FIGURE 2.   Design of the Atlanta Public Schools (APS) 8-center experiment.

The APS Study was an 8-center, 29-classroom experiment in which children were randomly assigned, within centers, to classrooms that differed systematically in level of staff education and staff/child ratio (Figure 2). Group size and caregiver experience were distributed as evenly as possible across the three experimental groups. Twelve of the experimental classrooms served 3-year-old children and 17 served 4-year-olds. This design made it possible to measure the main effects and interactions of staff education and staff/child ratio for children of different ages (3- and 4-year-olds).

Staff in the APS centers fell into three distinct categories of educational background. First, center directors (who were required to work in classrooms as well as to function as directors) had bachelor's degrees; most also had master's degrees. Second, lead teachers were graduates of the Atlanta Area Technical School (AAT) 2-year postsecondary training program in day care or had completed at least 2 years of college. Third, aides generally had high school diplomas (or an equivalent, such as the GED); the majority of aides had also completed the 60-hour, state-required training courses in day care offered through AAT. As shown in Figure 2, persons at these three levels of education were assigned to be lead teachers in the experimental APS classroom, some in classes with relatively high staff/child ratios, others in classes with lower ratios. Thus, ratio and education were crossed in a two-way factorial design. Children were then randomly assigned within centers to these experimentally organized classes. Random assignment, together with the fact that the children served by APS centers were unusually homogeneous in ethnic and socioeconomic background (virtually all were black children from low-income families) minimized any confounding of center characteristics and children's background characteristics.

The two Phase III components addressed similar questions, but had designs with different experimental strengths and weaknesses. Because the 49-center study included a large and diverse group of centers in three different sites, its results, if uniform across the sample, were likely to be widely generalizable; however, the diversity of the sample also posed challenges for analysis and interpretation. The APS study provided a greater degree of experimental control and afforded more safeguards against confounding of center characteristics with characteristics of the children, families, or communities served. However, the generalizability of its results was potentially limited by the homogeneity of the sample. The relatively consistent results actually obtained from the two study components constitute a sounder basis for policy conclusions that would findings from either component alone.

Variables and Measures

Choice of independent and dependent variables was motivated by a basic value decision made at the outset of the study by the funding agency and concurred with by its contractors, namely, the decision to focus attention on those aspects of the quality of day care that bear directly on the child. In effect, the funding agency and its contractors took the position that the primary goal of day care purchasing standards is to ensure the best possible environment for the most children. Other goals of day care, e.g., freeing parents to work, serving as a vehicle for delivery of social services to parents, employing low-income people as staff and fostering their development as professionals, were recognized as legitimate and important, but were not central to the study.

Independent Variables and Measures

Independent variables were of two types: background variables, such as age, sex, and race of children; socioeconomic characteristics of families and of the community served by the particular center; and policy variables, i.e., center characteristics subject to regulatory control. While background variables are unregulatable and, therefore, not of direct policy relevance, their effects had to be taken into account in assessing the effects of the policy variables.

Background variables.   Information on background characteristics of children and their families was gathered through interviews with parents. Background information included family income, sources of income, parents' education and occupation, length of parents' employment, number of siblings, and number of adults living in the house. Age, sex, and race of children were verified. In addition, census data were used to provide background information on demographic characteristics of the community, chiefly its socioeconomic and racial composition.

Policy variables.   As indicated earlier, the major policy variables examined in the NDCS fell into two categories, those relating to classroom composition and those relating to caregiver qualifications. Three variables fell under the rubric of classroom composition:

—*number of caregivers*, defined as the total number of caregivers present in or assigned to a classroom or group of children;[3]

—*group size*, defined as the total number of children present in or assigned to a class or to a principally responsible caregiver;[4] and

—*staff/child ratio*, defined as the number of caregivers divided by group size.

Information on variables related to classroom composition was gathered by two methods, one based on schedule or roster data and the other on direct observation. Schedule-based and observation-based measures of classroom composition were not always in close agreement. Differences between the two were primarily attributable to two phenomena: absenteeism and merging of classes. Because observations capture the group configurations actually experienced by the child and because they automatically take account of absenteeism and merging, observation-based measures were used in all analyses reported here. Three sets of observation-based data on classroom composition were collected. One set of counts was made in conjunction with behavioral observations of caregivers, and a second in conjunction with observations of children. These counts were used in the corresponding behavioral analyses. (Behavioral observations are described below.) A third set was collected on a regular basis by NDCS staff employed full-time at each center during Phases II and III. This set was used in analyses of children's gains on standardized tests, which were expected to reflect classroom configurations prevailing over the year, rather than at any particular point in time.

Group sizes in the study classrooms ranged from 8 to 36, with a mean of 17.6. Numbers of caregivers ranged from 1 to 5, with a mean of 2.4. Ratios ranged from 1:4 to 1:14, with a mean of 1:6.8.

Information on caregiver qualifications was gathered through interviews with nearly all caregivers who worked in the study's target classrooms, those serving primarily 3- and 4-year-old children. In assessing the relationship between caregiver qualifications and caregiver behavior (which used the individual caregiver—teacher or aide—as the unit of analysis), the qualifications of the individual in question were used directly as independent variables. In assessing effects on child behavior, qualifications of teachers and aides within each classroom were averaged together, and classes were the units of analysis. In assessing effects on children's test scores, qualifications of lead teachers, not aides, were averaged at the center level, and centers were the units of analysis.

Education levels of caregivers ranged from less than a high school diploma to graduate degrees; the mean number of years of education was 13.8. Experience ranged from none to many years; the average caregiver had 9 months of experience in day care prior to her current job, and 2 years and 9 months of experience in her current center.

Dependent Variables and Measures

Choosing dependent variables and measures to capture the child's experiences in the classroom and assess consequent changes in the child's development was perhaps the most challenging conceptual and practical task facing the NDCS. At the outset of the study, there existed no universally accepted catalogue of desirable experiences, traits, skills, and behaviors, nor does such a catalogue exist now. Even when the desirability of some experience or outcome was widely agreed upon in principle, adequate measures often did not exist. For example, there is fairly widespread agreement that an ideal care environment should build a child's self-concept, but satisfactory instruments for measuring the various aspects of self-concept in preschoolers have not yet been developed by basic researchers.

After a long process of experimentation and adjustment, chronicled in reports issued at the ends of Phase I and Phase II (Stallings,

Wilcox, & Travers, 1976; Travers, Coelen, & Ruopp, 1977), an empirical strategy of measurement and analysis evolved. The strategy relied heavily on two observation instruments selected in Phase I. Of the two instruments, one focused on caregivers and one on children. Both used trained, on-site observers to record everyday classroom behavior in considerable detail. From the resulting records of frequencies of specific behaviors, measures of broader variables were constructed, usually by summing frequencies of behaviors that were conceptually related and empirically correlated. In addition, two standardized tests designed to measure selected school-related cognitive and linguistic skills were administered to each child. In short, the study attempted to describe as objectively and comprehensively as possible the behaviors associated with various configurations of regulated center characteristics and to supplement this information with information about children's test performance. The study's conclusions and policy recommendations rest on largely post hoc value judgements about the total pattern of caregiver behavior, child behavior, and test scores found to be associated with the different regulatory variables. Further details on variables and measures in the three domains are provided immediately below.

Caregiver behavior. Variables in the domain of caregiver behavior primarily characterize the nature and number of contacts between caregivers and children. The variables distinguish warm, stimulating child-directed behavior from more passive and instrumental forms of behavior. They also distinguish interaction directed at individual children and small groups from interaction directed at larger groups and other adults. Variables in this domain include:

—social interaction with children (praising, comforting, responding, questioning, and instructing);
—management of children (commanding and correcting);
—observing children;
—center-related activities (planning, arranging materials, cleanup, recordkeeping, etc.);
—overall frequencies of all types of interactions with individual children, small groups (2–7 children), medium groups (8–12 children), large groups (13 or more children), and other adults.

The system used to measure these variables, the SRI Preschool Observation Instrument, also called the Adult-Focus Instrument

(AFI), was a modification of a system originally developed by Jane Stallings of SRI International to evaluate follow through classrooms (Stallings, 1975). Stallings altered the system for the NDCS to record adult behaviors in day care centers. The AFI consists of a Physical Environment Inventory, which describes space, materials, and equipment in the classroom; a Classroom Snapshot, which describes general activity patterns at a point in time; and a Five-Minute Interaction record, which describes the behavior of a particular caregiver in detail. Frequencies of behaviors recorded in the Five-Minute Interaction records were used to construct the variables listed above. Reliabilities, or "generalizabilities," of AFI behavior codes, such as "praise" and "command," and of broader constructs, such as "social interaction," were calculated using techniques developed by Cronbach and his colleagues (Cronbach, Gleser, Nanda, & Rejaratnam, 1972). Generalizabilities were in the .4–.7 range for individual codes and were well over .8 for broader constructs. Caregivers were observed in both Fall 1976 and Spring 1977. There were 220 caregivers: approximately ⅔ lead teachers and ⅓ aides. They were observed at each time point.

   Child behavior. Variables in the domain of child behavior characterize both the child's social interactions and solitary activities, as well as relative amounts of interaction with adults, other children, and objects in the physical environment. The variables distinguish activities of a verbal/intellectual and/or social nature from behavior indicating passivity or withdrawal. Variables in this domain include:

—verbal initiative (giving opinions, preferences, information, or comments);
—reflection/innovation (considering, contemplating, tinkering, or adding a new idea or new object to an ongoing activity);
—cooperation/compliance (active, appropriate responding to questions, requests, and commands from adults and other children);
—general interest/participation in center activities
—aimless wandering;
—noninvolvement in tasks in activities;
—task persistence (duration of longest activity in an observation period);
—attention to adults;
—attention to other children;
—attention to the environment.

The system used to measure these variables—the Prescott-SRI Child Observation System, or Child-Focus Instrument (CFI)—was an adaptation of a system designed specifically to assess day care environments (Prescott, Jones, Kritchevsky, Milich, & Haselhoef, 1975). Generalizabilities of CFI measures at the level of the individual child were very low. Generalizabilities of these measures when averaged to class level were still modest (ranging from .1 to .7, typically around .4), but in many cases, were adequate to support analysis. Thus, the variables are probably best regarded as descriptors of the social atmosphere of classrooms rather than as measures of individual traits. Consequently, analyses of child observation data were conducted using classes, not children, as units of analysis. Samples of approximately 1100 children (almost entirely overlapping) were observed in both Fall 1976 and Spring 1977. The number of classes observed at each time point was 145 (116 in the 49-center study and 29 in the APS study).

Test scores.   Variables in this domain were adjusted gains from fall to spring on two standardized tests: the Preschool Inventory (PSI), a global test of school-related skills and knowledge, including knowledge of shapes, sizes, parts of the body, spatial relationships, etc. and the Peabody Picture Vocabulary Test (PPVT), a measure of receptive vocabulary in which the child matches words and pictures. The tests were *not* assumed to measure general cognitive or linguistic ability or development; moreover, their cultural biases were acknowledged. They were included as outcome measures because of their potential for predicting the child's success in elementary school, a concern of many parents and providers. Fall-to-spring gains were calculated using techniques designed to circumvent certain well-known technical problems involved in measuring change (See Goodrich & Singer, 1980). Reliabilities of both tests exceeded .9 when administered at each time point. Reliabilities of change scores were approximately .6. Change scores were calculated for approximately 1100 children who were tested in both the fall and spring.

Results

The Phase III Experiments

Results of the Phase III experiments suggest that the regulatory variables chosen for experimental manipulation, primarily staff/ child ratio and secondarily staff education, have few detectable effects on the behavior of caregivers, the behavior of children, or children's test scores. ANOVA's using the various experimental conditions as classificatory variables revealed only widely scattered significant relationships to the dependent variables listed earlier. High staff/child ratios did appear to have some positive effects, but these effects were neither consistent nor large and may have been due to chance.

There were, however, some differences involving the staff/child ratios, but these were not due to experimental manipulation.

Within each of the various experimental groups of centers and classes, there was a great deal of variation, not only in the experimentally manipulated variables (ratio and staff education), but also in other nonexperimental regulatable characteristics (group size, staff experience, and child-related content of caregivers' education or training). These naturally occurring variations were examined, through multiple regression analysis, in relation to the dependent variables listed earlier. In a general sense, these analyses confirmed the experimental results already reported that variations in staff/child ratio (within the range studied in the NDCS) have some effects, but fewer than generally believed, and that the formal education of caregivers is a relatively unimportant influence on the child's experience in day care and his or her test performance. However, other regulatable center characteristics, notably, group size and education or training in fields specifically related to young children, did show important relationships to outcomes for children.

Classroom Composition and Caregiver Behavior

It is in the domain of caregiver behavior that the effects of group size were least clear and the effects of staff/child ratio strongest. However, the effects of high ratios (few children per caregiver) were not uniformly positive from the child's point of view.

Analyses of effects of classroom composition on caregiver behavior were clouded by atypically high collinearity between group size and staff/child ratio. On-site counts of adults and children taken in tandem with the caregiver observations yielded a correlation between group size and ratio of about .45. Thus, effects of ratio and group size could not always be clearly separated. In particular, where groups were large and/or ratios low (many children per caregiver), lead caregivers spent a relatively large portion of their time observing children passively rather than interacting with them. Also, in large and/or low-ratio classes, lead caregivers tended to deal with children collectively, in clusters of 13 or more, rather than in small groups of 2–7. In general, however, correlations between independent variables ranged from zero to about .25, so that multiple regression analyses using combinations of background and policy variables were not much threatened by multicollinearity.

It should be pointed out, however, that staff/child ratios did show some relationships to caregiver behavior that were not found for group size. High ratios appeared to make management of children easier; caregivers spent less time commanding and correcting children in high ratio classes. Also, in high-ratio classes, adults spent more time with other adults and in activities not involving children, such as performance of routine chores (center-related activity). This outcome may suggest that high ratios benefit caregivers by providing contact with other adults and time to do necessary tasks, but it also suggests that in high-ratio classes, some of the time potentially available for children is diverted to activities in which children are not directly involved.

Classroom Composition and Child Behavior

Children in small groups showed higher frequencies of cooperation and compliance and of reflection and innovation (considering, contemplating, contributing new ideas) than children in large groups. They also showed a marginal tendency to engage in more verbal initiative (giving opinions, making spontaneous comments). Aimless wandering and lack of involvement in tasks or activities were less common among children in small groups than among those in larger groups. (Separate analyses, not discussed in detail here, also showed that threats, squabbles, and hostility, while rare in all NDCS child observations, were especially rare in small groups.) These relationships between classroom composition and child behavior are illustrated in Figure 3. Panels A and B illustrate the progressive decline in frequency of reflection/innovation and cooperation across groups of increasing size. Panels C and D illustrate the progressive increase in frequency of noninvolvement and aimless wandering in groups of increasing size. The sloping lines in the figure represent simple least-squares regressions of designated behaviors on group size. However, all relationships shown in this and later figures were established through numerous multivariate tests. Shaded areas in the figure, between group sizes of 12 and 24, represent the region in which 75% of NDCS classrooms lie. Curved lines represent 95% confidence bands around the regression line. Data are shown for classrooms in the 49-center sample in Spring 1977 (N=87). Again, however, results are shown only if they were fairly consistently observed in other data sets.

Group size also affected broader patterns of interaction shown by the child. In smaller groups, children devoted more of their attention to adults; in larger groups, they tended more to interact with other children collectively. These relationships are illustrated in Figure 4.

Links between staff/child ratio and child behavior were not as consistent across data sets as those between group size and child behavior. In the spring 49-center data, children in high-ratio classes showed more interest, participation, and task persistence than their counterparts in low-ratio centers. However, because these relationships were not found in either the APS data or the fall 49-center data, this cannot be declared with confidence.

It is significant that high ratios were not associated with the overall frequency of child-adult interaction. The principal rationale for use of ratio as a regulatory tool has been that high ratios allow caregivers more time for each individual child. Earlier it was reported that lead teachers spend some of this additional time with other adults and in center-related activity. Apparently, enough of the caregiver's time is devoted to these activities to nullify the potential increase in adult-child interaction made possible by high ratios. It is significant that total group size, unlike ratio, *is* associated with child-adult interaction.

Classroom Composition and Gains on the PSI and PPVT

As indicated earlier, NDCS analyses of test scores focused on children's fall-to-spring gains on the PSI and PPVT. The gain scores used in the analysis were not simple differences of spring and fall scores, but adjusted values calculated to avoid certain technical problems posed by simple difference scores. These adjusted gain scores were found to have two extremely important properties. They were almost completely independent of the child's age, sex, race, family income, mother's education, and other socio-economic background characteristics.[5] Moreover, they were relatively independent of the racial and socioeconomic composition of the center as a whole. These properties were important in that they made further statistical adjustments to compensate for effects of socioeconomic and demographic background variables much less critical than they might otherwise have been.

A. REFLECTION/INNOVATION

NUMBER OF TIMES
(and percent of total observation time)
OBSERVED PER HOUR at 12 second intervals

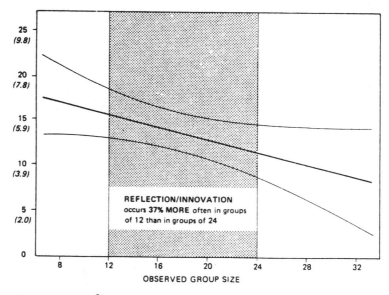

B. COOPERATION [a]

NUMBER OF TIMES
(and percent of total observation time)
OBSERVED PER HOUR at 12 second intervals

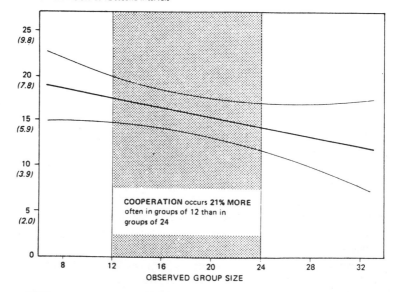

FIGURE 3.   Relationships between child behavior and group size.

C. NONINVOLVEMENT

NUMBER OF TIMES
(and percent of total observation time)
OBSERVED PER HOUR at 12 second intervals

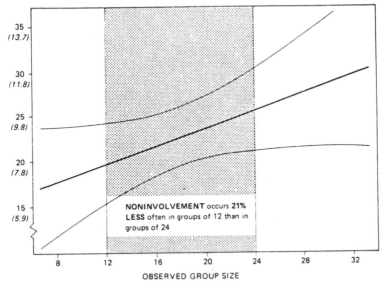

NONINVOLVEMENT occurs **21%
LESS** often in groups of 12 than in
groups of 24

OBSERVED GROUP SIZE

D. AIMLESS WANDERING

NUMBER OF TIMES
(and percent of total observation time)
OBSERVED PER HOUR at 12 second intervals

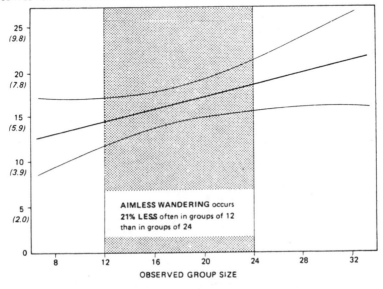

AIMLESS WANDERING occurs
21% LESS often in groups of 12
than in groups of 24

OBSERVED GROUP SIZE

(FIGURE 3. continued)

A. ATTENTION TO GROUPS

NUMBER OF TIMES
(and percent of total observation time)
OBSERVED PER HOUR at 12 second intervals

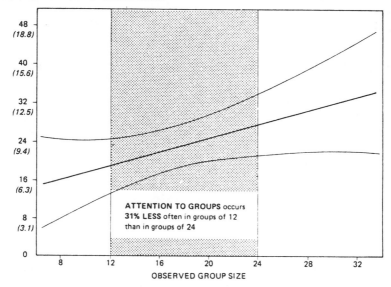

ATTENTION TO GROUPS occurs
31% LESS often in groups of 12
than in groups of 24

OBSERVED GROUP SIZE

B. ATTENTION TO ADULTS

NUMBER OF TIMES
(and percent of total observation time)
OBSERVED PER HOUR at 12 second intervals

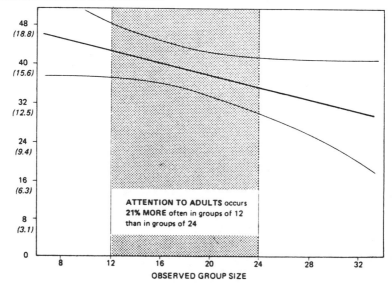

ATTENTION TO ADULTS occurs
21% MORE often in groups of 12
than in groups of 24

OBSERVED GROUP SIZE

FIGURE 4.   Relationship between object of child's attention and group size.

Children's gains on the PSI were higher in centers that maintained smaller groups of children (and caregivers) than in centers with larger groups. For example, gains averaged approximately 7.0 points in groups of 12 children, compared to 5.9 points in groups of 24. The difference of 1.1 points represents a 19% advantage in growth rate in groups of 12 compared to groups of 24. Since children's gains averaged about 6.5 points over the 7-month period between fall and spring (about .9 points per month), the 1.1 point difference also translates into 1.2 months differential gain over the 7-month period in groups of 12 compared to groups of 24. (Most children in the sample gained more rapidly than children tested in previous national studies; the difference between small and large groups corresponds to almost two months' gain in these earlier studies.) Similarly, gains on the PPVT were 1.7 points higher in groups of 12 children over a 7-month period than in groups of 24, a 23% acceleration in growth in small groups as opposed to large groups, corresponding to roughly 1.6 months differential gain in a 7-month period. The relationship between group size and test score gains is illustrated in Figure 5, which parallels previous figures except that centers (N=57) rather than classrooms are the units of interest.[6] By contrast, no significant relationships were found between staff/child ratio and gains on the PSI or PPVT.

Effects of Caregiver Qualifications

As indicated earlier, the NDCS examined correlates of four components of caregiver qualifications: (1) years of formal education, regardless of subject matter or specialization; (2) presence or absence of specialized preparation relevant to young children, obtained either within a formal degree program or in a training program unrelated to any degree; (3) amount of day care work experience prior to the caregiver's beginning work at her/his current center; and (4) length of service in the current center. The results can be summarized as follows: Amount of formal education, without regard for content, showed only a few scattered relationships to child and caregiver behavior and bore no detectable relationship to test score gains. In contrast, education/training in child-related fields such as developmental psychology, day care, early childhood education, or special education was associated with distinctive patterns of caregiver and child behavior and with higher gains in test scores for children. These patterns roughly parallelled those associated with small groups, though

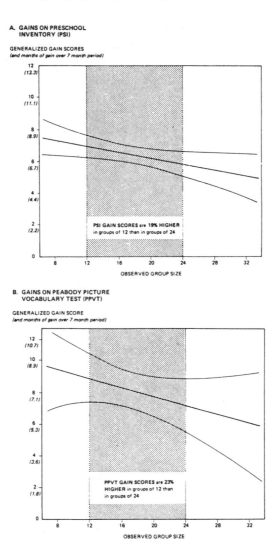

Shaded portions of figures, between group sizes of 12 and 24, correspond to the region in which the middle 75 percent of NDCS centers lie.

FIGURE 5.   Relationship between child's test score gains and group size.

they were not as strong or as widespread. Results for experience were inconclusive.

Lead teachers with specialized education or training engaged in substantially more social interaction with children (questioning, instructing, responding, praising, and comforting) than caregivers without such education or training. This relationship is illustrated in Figure 6.[7]

SOCIAL INTERACTION

NUMBER OF TIMES
(and percent of total observation time)
OBSERVED PER HOUR at 5 second intervals

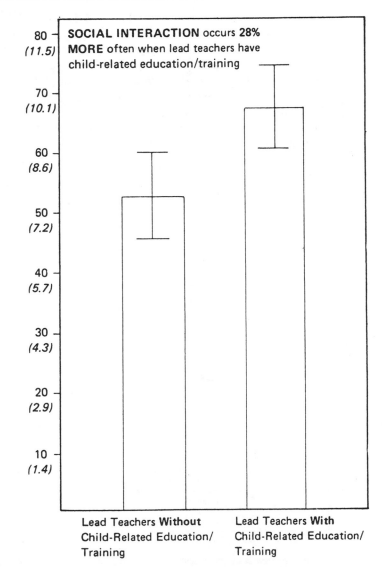

CHILD-RELATED EDUCATION/TRAINING

FIGURE 6: Relationship between lead teacher behavior and lead teacher child-related education/training.

Children in classes led by caregivers with specialized preparation showed more cooperation and compliance and were less frequently uninvolved in tasks or activities than children in other classes. They also showed longer durations of attention to tasks or activities.

Test score gains were also affected by caregivers' child-related training, as shown in Figure 7.[8] Children in centers where all of the caregivers had child-related preparation gained 1.4 more points on the PSI from fall to spring than did children in centers where no caregivers had such preparation, a 25% advantage in growth rate for children in the former group, corresponding to a differential gain of 1.5 months over a 7-month period.

Finally, day care experience showed some effects in all three dependent domains—caregiver behavior, child behavior, and test scores. However, as was the case for education, these relationships were inconsistent across data sets and are not readily interpretable. Many of the effects of experience were confined to a few centers

**GAINS ON THE PRESCHOOL
INVENTORY (PSI)**

GENERALIZED GAIN SCORES
(and months of gain over 7 month period)

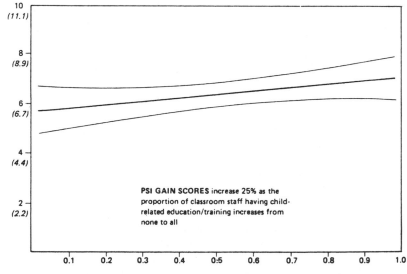

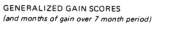

PROPORTION OF CLASSROOM STAFF WITH CHILD-RELATED EDUCATION/TRAINING

FIGURE 7.   Relationship between child PSI gains and classroom staff child-related education/training (center average).

where staff had worked in day care for a very long time. With these centers excluded from the sample, many effects of experience disappeared.

Relationship between Formal Education and Child-Related Specialization

An important policy question related to the above findings is whether child-related training is effective for individuals with little formal education and, if so, what kind of training works best. Unfortunately, the study sample was not adequate to address these issues.

Many caregivers in the sample who had specialized in child-related areas did so in the context of a program of postsecondary education. Some, however, received their training in the context of a high school program, and a number of caregivers in Atlanta took a state-required 60-hour training course after high school but outside of any formal degree program. Most of these programs involved substantial amounts of practical field training coupled with varying amounts of classroom training.

It would have been illuminating to compare subsamples of caregivers with little formal education, some with and some without specific types of child-related training. However, it was not possible to identify appropriate subsamples of sufficient size for statistical analysis. Thus, it was not possible to determine whether child-related training is effective specifically for caregivers with little formal education. Similarly, it proved impossible to identify subsamples that could be used to distinguish effects for the practical field component of this training from the classroom component, nor was it possible to single out any particular curriculum or training approach as particularly valuable.

Interchangeability of Education, Experience, and Training

A second policy issue, on which NDCS findings do throw some light, concerns the interchangeability of education, experience, and child-related training as avenues for preparation of competent caregivers. The 1968 FIDCR stipulate that "educational activities must be under the supervision and direction of a staff member trained or experienced in child growth and development," implying that training and experience are in some sense equivalent routes to competence. Many state regulations likewise imply interchangeability of training and experience or of education and experience. Often, educational requirements are framed in terms of degrees or diplomas without regard for major area of study. NDCS data indicate rather clearly that neither education in fields unrelated to children nor day care experience per se is equivalent to child-related education/training.

Interactions Between Classroom Composition and Caregiver Qualifications

Another important issue to consider in framing child care regulations is whether optimum group structures and optimum caregiver qualifications can be specified independently or whether they are mutually contingent. For example, consider whether the optimum group size is the same for caregivers with or without education or training in a child-related field. Both of these variables, taken separately, contribute to quality in child care. However, it might be the case that caregivers with child-related education/training can effectively handle groups of widely varying size, while less qualified caregivers are effective only with smaller groups. (Such a situation would appear in the data as a statistical interaction involving child-related education/training and group-size.) Alternatively, it might be the case that all caregivers, with and without appropriate training or education, are more effective with smaller groups, and that qualified caregivers are more effective than others with groups of any size.

The statistical power of the NDCS to detect interaction effects was limited. Unless such effects were large, they could not have been detected within the constraints of the sample size. Subject to these limitations, no consistent interactions between composition and qualifications variables were found. Thus, the most prudent conclusion to be drawn from NDCS data on interactions is that classroom composition and caregiver qualifications contribute independently to quality. Benefits to children appear to be greatest when classroom composition and staff qualifications are both set at the optimum practically achievable levels.

Conclusions and Policy Recommendations

Perhaps the most general and important finding of the study was that variations in regulatable center characteristics do make a difference in the well-being of children. In contrast to many earlier studies of the effects of variations in curriculum or resource outlay in education, the NDCS showed clearly that it matters how day care classes are arranged and who staffs them. To be sure, much of what goes on in day care is *not* influenced by regulatable center characteristics. There is a great deal of variability in the quality of human interaction in day care settings even when the composition of the classroom and the qualifications of caregivers are fixed. Nevertheless, regulatable characteristics, particularly group size and child-related education/training of caregivers, show relationships to measures of children's experience and of developmental change that are significant both statistically and substantively.

Because the results of the NDCS are essentially correlational, they do not permit strict causal inferences. It can be stated with some confidence that group size and child-related education/training are associated with positive aspects of the social environment in day care and with superior test performance of children. It is a plausible but unproven conjecture that changing existing practices through regulation and other policy tools (e.g., providing funds for training of caregivers) will produce the same desirable effects. Nevertheless, even if causality cannot be inferred with certainty, the study's findings are useful in setting purchasing standards. Because small groups and appropriately trained caregivers are reliably associated with aspects of quality, they can be used as benchmarks for selecting centers in which the government will buy care, even if they are not in themselves causes of positive outcomes.

To arrive at policy recommendations, the findings reported above were integrated with results from other components of the study which were concerned with the costs associated with the various regulatable center characteristics and with prevailing practices in staffing and group composition among centers nationally. The costs of maintaining small groups and of employing staff trained or educated in child-related fields were found to be small, whereas the costs associated with maintaining high staff/child ratios were significant. Consequently, it was recommended that, for preschoolers, the group size standards of the existing FIDCR be maintained or made more stringent, while the ratio requirements be relaxed slightly. The expected result would be an improvement in the quality of care for preschoolers, together with a reduction in costs relative to those that would prevail if the Title XX FIDCR were enforced. Implementation of the NDCS recommendations would not require major disruption of current practice, since a high proportion of centers nationally already maintain both relatively small groups and staff/child ratios that are only a little less stringent than those mandated by the FIDCR,[9] despite claims of some providers and state Title XX administrators that the FIDCR ratios are unrealistically strict.

For infants and toddlers, institution of a group size standard and maintenance of the current ratio standard were recommended. (Findings of the infant/toddler substudy suggested that for these younger children, in contrast to 3- to 5-year-olds, ratio was an important determinant of quality.) It was also recommended that training or education in a child-related field be required of all individuals providing direct care to children and that states be required to make such training available.

As indicated, many elements of these recommendations were adopted by HEW when it proposed new day care regulations early in 1980. Whether they will be incorporated into law by Congress remains to be seen. Regardless of the final outcome, the process by which HEW's proposed regulations were developed represents an encouraging attempt at integrating social values, political factors, and the findings of applied social science in policy determination.

FOOTNOTES

1. The Title XX FIDCR require ratios of 1 adult to 4 children for ages 6 weeks to 3 years, 1:5 for 3-year-olds in groups no larger than 15, and 1:7 for 4-year-olds in groups no larger than 20. On the average, the states allow ratios of 1:11.4 for 3-year-olds and 1:13.7 for 4-year-olds.

2. In conformance with HEW directives, manipulations consisted only of making low ratios higher. The Group I treatment simulates one potential effect of full enforcement of FIDCR under Title XX, namely, an increase in ratios in centers serving publicly funded children, but currently operating below FIDCR ratios.

3. In all but a few NDCS centers, groups of children were assigned to particular rooms, supervised by a single caregiver or several caregivers. In a few "open classroom" centers, however, very large numbers of children (approaching 100 in extreme cases) were present in a single large room. Even in such centers, children clustered around individual caregivers or small teams dispersed around the room, though children were often free to move from group to group. Numbers of children in these smaller groups constituted the group sizes used for NDCS analytic purposes. Similarly, numbers of caregivers were the number of adults in physically separated groups.

4. In day care classrooms, unlike most public school classrooms, it is not usual to find a single adult in charge. Configurations of two or three caregivers, usually a teacher plus aides, are more common. Both the number of children and the number of adults varies significantly from classroom to classroom. It is for this reason that staff/child ratio and group size can vary more or less independently and must be examined separately. It cannot simply be assumed that large classes will have low ratios, nor that small classes will have high ratios.

5. As expected, on the basis of results of other studies, there was a slight influence of race on PPVT gain scores. However, the effect was so small, it had virtually no analytic consequences. PPVT scores were nevertheless statistically adjusted prior to analyses to remove the minor difference associated with race.

6. Meaningful analyses of class-average changes on the PSI and PPVT could not be conducted because children changed classes and because classes frequently split or merged between fall and spring. Therefore, analyses of test scores were conducted using both the individual child and the whole center as units of analyses. Note that instability of class membership did not affect class-level analyses of behavioral data, reported above, since no change measures were involved.

7. The figure is a bar graph rather than a line because there are only two possible conditions: Lead teachers either have or do not have child-related education/training. The "I"-shaped marker at the top of each bar represents the 95% confidence interval, corresponding to the thin curving lines in all other graphs. Reported results focus on lead teachers rather than aides, because too few aides have child-related training to permit meaningful comparisons among aides.

8. Children's behavior and test score gains were examined in relation to the proportion of all caregivers in each classroom or center who had child-related education/training. Though the variable has only two possible values for each individual caregiver, it can take many values across the range from zero to one for a class or center, because there are different mixes of caregiver preparation within classes or centers. Both teachers and aides were included in calculations for classes and centers, because children's behavior and test score gains are presumably affected by all of the caregivers to whom children are exposed.

9. Staff/child ratios nationwide, averaging over all classes and ages of children, are 1:6.8, compared to 1:6.3 required by the FIDCR and 1:12.5 permitted by state licensing requirement (Coelen, Glantz, & Calore, 1978).

REFERENCES

Belsky, J., & Steinberg, L. D. The effects of day care: A critical review. *Child Development*, 1978, *49*, 929–949.
Coelen, C., Glantz, F., & Calore, D. *Day care centers in the U.S.: A national profile 1976–1977. Final report of the national day care study* (Vol. III). Cambridge, MA: Abt Books, 1978.
Congressional Budget Office. *Childcare and preschool: Options for federal support.* Washington, D.C.: U.S. Government Printing Office, 1978.
Cronbach, L. J., Gleser, G. C., Nanda, H., & Rajaratnam, N. *The dependability of behavioral measures: Theory of generalizability for scores and profiles.* New York: Wiley, 1972.
Etaugh, C. Effects of nonmaternal care on children. *American Psychologist*, 1980, *35*, 309–319.
Federal Register, March 19, 1980.
Fraiberg, S. *Every child's birthright: In defense of mothering.* New York: Basic Books, 1977.
Goodrich, R., & Singer, J. Analysis of test score growth in the national day care study. In N. Goodrich (Ed.), *National day care study effects analyses. Final report of the national day care study* (Vol. IV-C). Cambridge, MA: Abt Books, 1980.
Prescott, E., Jones, E., Kritchevsky, S., Milich, C., & Haselhoef, E. *Assessment of child-rearing environments: An ecological approach.* Pasadena, CA: Pacific Oaks College, 1975.
Ruopp, R., Travers, J., Glantz, F., & Coelen, C. *Children at the center. Final report of the national day care study* (Vol. I). Cambridge, MA: Abt Books, 1979.
Stallings, J. Implementation and child effects of teaching practices in follow through classrooms. *Monographs of the Society for Research in Child Development*, 1975, *40*, (7–8, Serial No. 163).
Stallings, J., Wilcox, M., & Travers, J. *Phase II instruments for the National day care cost-effects study: Instrument selection and field testing.* Menlo Park, CA: SRI International, 1976.

Travers, J., Coelen, C., & Ruopp, R. *National Day care study second annual report 1975–1976: Phase II results and phase III design.* Cambridge, MA: Abt Associates, 1977.
Travers, J., Goodson, B. D., Singer, J., & Connell, D. *Research results of the National Day Care Study. Final report of the national day care study* (Vol. II). Cambridge, MA: Abt Books, 1980.

THE PROBLEM-SOLVING APPROACH TO ADJUSTMENT: A COMPETENCY-BUILDING MODEL OF PRIMARY PREVENTION

Myrna B. Shure
George Spivack

ABSTRACT. Social maladjustment is, to a significant extent, a function of an individual's inability to effectively identify and solve problems of an interpersonal life situation. The Interpersonal Cognitive Problem Solving (ICPS) training approach was developed to enhance social adjustment and interpersonal competence by increasing one's interpersonal problem solving abilities. Emphasis is placed on enhancing the trainee's ability to: (a) generate problem solutions (b) determine suitable means of achieving end goals, while (c) recognizing the consequences of alternate strategies. Research results and program evaluation indicate the validity and viability of this approach for children as young as 4 and 5 years of age.

There are lots of ways to affect behavior and enhance the social competence of young children. We can advise or suggest strategies of action. We can reward what we deem to be positive behaviors and punish those thought to be negative. We can reason, model, and offer choices. All of these techniques, however, add up to one thing: we are doing the thinking for the child. Our approach is different. We believe that even very young children can, or can learn to, think for themselves and solve everyday interpersonal problems. Those who can do this are likely to be better adjusted than those who cannot.

Think for themselves. Better adjusted. This linkage is derived from a decade of research with individuals across a wide variety of

The authors' problem-solving research for 4- and 5-year-olds was supported in part by Grant No. MH-20372, 1971–1975; research with 10-year-olds, by Grant No. MH-27741, 1978–1979, Life Course Review Committee (formerly Applied Research Branch), National Institute of Mental Health. Reprints may be requested from Myrna B. Shure, Department of Mental Health Sciences, Hahnemann Medical College, 112 North Broad Street, Philadelphia, PA 19102.

age groups, in various social class and ethnic groups, and across a
wide range of general intellectual abilities. The underlying problem-
solving approach for all those groups has been an attempt to
identify processes that are central to social adjustment. By understanding the processes, training programs can be implemented to
help individuals better manage life's interpersonal stresses. To
appreciate the quality of human adjustment, one must understand
what allows one person to grow up in and maneuver through the
interpersonal arena with reasonable self-esteem and confidence,
while another does not. Probably no theory of human adjustment
of psychopathology exists wherein quality of social relationships
and ability to cope with other people are not at the core of things.
Our earlier work with the middle class and the poor, including
children, adolescents, and adults, has shown that regardless of IQ,
there is a key determinant of the quality of social adjustment, a set
of mediating skills that define one's capacity to think through and
solve interpersonal problems (Spivack, 1973; Spivack, Platt, &
Shure, 1976). These mediating skills involve not *what* one thinks,
but *how* one thinks when confronted with an interpersonal problem
situation. While content specificity is not irrelevant, the primary
issue is the state or process of thought.

One such interpersonal cognitive problem-solving (ICPS) skill
is the capacity to generate alternative solutions to interpersonal
problems. This would seem to closely parallel group brainstorming,
wherein people offer a variety of possible solutions. Judgement
and censorship are, however, suspended. The key feature is that of
generating different solution possibilities. The individual man-
ifests this skill by demonstrating an ability to draw different
categories of solution to a given problem. The process involves how
much the person thinks in terms of options: "I could do this or that,
or I could even do that . . . ." In contrast, the individual scoring low
on the alternative solutions skill testing characteristically fore-
closes thought without considering alternative routes.

As reviewed in Spivack, Platt, and Shure (1976), this alternative solution skill relates to adjustment across a wide range of age
groups: preschoolers, 10-year-olds, adolescents, adults, and, more
recently discovered, in individuals in their 70s and 80s (Spivack,
Standen, Bryson, & Garrett, Note 1). It is the most important skill
we have yet studied among 4- and 5-year-olds. It differentiates
normal from inhibited and shy, as well as from impulsive children.

A second ICPS skill related to adjustment involves considering
the consequences of one's social acts in terms of their impact both

on other people and on oneself. The process is one of pursuing the thought of an act to the point of asking "What might happen as a result of my doing this?" Under this rubric are categorized several kinds of thinking behavior. One involves whether a person *spontaneously* considers consequences when contemplating an action. Very often the individual who says, "I'm sorry for what I did—I just didn't think," is essentially saying that he/she knew what he/she wanted, but did not consider that he/she may be stepping on someone else's toes. A different type of consequential thinking involves the ability to generate *alternative* consequences. For example, a person might think "If I yell at him for what he did, he might better appreciate the seriousness of the matter, *or* he might only feel hurt and not really listen to me, *or* he might not be my friend when I need him . . ." and so forth.

The spontaneous tendency to consider social consequences does not become important for adjustment until adolescence. This is not to say that young children cannot think this way, rather, this process does not seem to play a crucial role in early social adjustment. Recent studies with elderly people (Spivack et al., Note 1) also suggest that this skill is least likely to deteriorate with old age.

In contrast to spontaneous consequential thinking, the ability to generate alternative consequences to a given act becomes significant for social adjustment quite early in life. Among 4-year-olds, for example, alternative consequential ability differentiates between overly impulsive and overly inhibited children. Impulsive youngsters are less able than normal youngsters to generate alternative solutions to problems, but do generate alternative consequences fairly well. Impulsive children may repeatedly get into difficulty even if they know the consequences of their actions, because often they cannot think of what else to do (Spivack & Shure, 1974; Shure & Spivack, Note 2).

A third ICPS skill is that of articulating the step-by-step means that are necessary in order to carry out the solution to any interpersonal problem. This spelling out of the so-called means-end often incorporates recognition of obstacles that must be overcome and an appreciation that reaching a goal may take time. Means-ends thinking may be viewed as a defining of an interpersonal road map that lays out in some detail how one may proceed in solving an interpersonal problem.

Means-ends thinking emerges as significant for adjustment in public school children between ages 8 and 10 (Shure & Spivack, 1972), a finding recently confirmed by Pelligrini (Note 3), and remains so throughout adulthood (Platt & Spivack, 1973; Platt, Spivack, Altman, Altman, & Peizer, 1974) and into old age (Spivack, et al., Note 1). Such thinking has been shown to be deficient in individuals exhibiting a wide range of social problems. Means-ends thought has been found to be more deficient in psychiatric groups than normals (Coché, Note 4), more deficient in delin-quents than nondelinquents (Spivack & Levine, Note 5), more deficient in depressed than nondepressed college students (Gotlib & Asarnow, 1979), more deficient in teenagers with unwanted pregnancies than those without (Steinlauf, 1979), and more defi-cient in poor adjusting than better adjusting drug abusers in rehabilitation programs (Appel, Kaestner, & Sofer, Note 6).

Having identified three processes of ICPS thinking that are clearly associated with quality of social adjustment, the critical issue becomes whether enhancing these skills through training can play a key role in diminishing observable behavioral difficulties and maladaption and/or in increasing positive coping strategies when interpersonal difficulties arise. Such training has been and is being conducted in a variety of settings for a variety of age groups. Examples include lower SES preschoolers (Allen, 1978; Shure & Spivack, Note 2), middle SES preschoolers (Wowkanech, Note 7), hyperaggressive 7-year-olds (Camp & Bash, Note 8), urban and suburban elementary school aged children (Allen, Chinsky, Larcen, Lockman, & Selinger, 1976; Bensky, 1978; Elardo & Cald-well, 1979; Elias, 1978; Enright, 1980; McClure, Chinsky & Larcen, 1978; Weissberg, Geston, Rapkin, Boike, Cowen, Davidson, Flores de Apodaca, McKim, & Rains, Note 9), retarded-educable 6- to 12-year-olds (Healey, 1977), young adult alcohol abusers (Intagli-ata, 1978), adult psychiatric patients (Coché, Note 4), child abus-ers (Nesbitt-Brown, Note 10), and drug abusers (Platt, Morell, & Flaherty, Note 11).

In this paper, one specific set of programs will be discussed, programs designed by the authors for teachers and parents of inner-city, lower socioeconomic level, 4- and 5-year-old children. They were developed on the basis of having identified, through correlational research, those ICPS skills most significantly re-lated to social adjustment before training. Following a description of the programs, findings will be discussed in light of implications for primary prevention, followed by a section on some of the practi-cal and scientific difficulties in performing rigorous evaluation of this kind of intervention.

The Training Programs

The format of the nursery program is a script (Spivack & Shure, 1974; Shure & Spivack, Note 12), upgraded in sophistication for use in kindergarten (Shure & Spivack, Note 13) and modified for flexible use with a single child at home (Shure & Spivack, 1978). Children are exposed to 3 months of daily 20-minutes lessons in game form, beginning with simple word concepts built in for later association in problem solving. For example, the word *not* is taught so children can later decide what and what not to do and whether an idea is or is not a good one. The word *or* helps children think about the idea that there is more than one way to solve a problem: "I can do this or I can do that." The word *different* helps one to later think of different things to do. Identification of and sensitivity to people's feelings is important in problem solving. Children learn that there is more than one way to find out how people feel and what they like by watching what they do, hearing what they say, and asking if they are not sure. To help children understand the effect of their behavior on others, and of others' behavior on them, games focus on why a child might feel as he does: "He's mad because I took his toy."

After mastery of these kinds of skills, generally in about 8 weeks, children are presented with pictures and puppets depicting interpersonal problem situations and are asked for all the ways they can think of for the portrayed child to, for example, "get another to let him help feed the hamsters." All solutions are accepted equally—forceful ones as "hit" or "grab the food," and nonforceful ones as "say please," "I'll be your friend," or offering a toy. In subsequent games, the children evaluate for themselves whether an idea is or is not a good one and why. Because it is the ability to generate multiple options more than content that relates to healthy adjustment, the idea is not to take away from poor problem solvers what they already know, but to help them think about what else they can do; to discover that there is more than one way to do things. Therefore, solutions are never reinforced for being good, but rather for being different.

Teachers were also helped to develop ways to talk with children when real problems came up, problem-solving techniques which were quite rewarding and later included as part of the mother's training as well. Before training, one teacher could not get Rochelle to stop grabbing toys from children:

> T: Rochelle, why do you keep grabbing the doll like that?
> C: It's mine. She won't let me hold it.
> T: You know not to take things. You're supposed to take turns.
> C: But . . .
> T: If you keep taking things, no one will play with you.
> C: I don't care, I want the doll.
> T: Then ask her nicely.

Although the teacher asked the child why she grabbed the toy, her intent was to teach the child what was important from her own point of view, not the child's. Instead of encouraging Rochelle to express the problem from her vantage point or to think of how to resolve it, the teacher only continued to explicate the adversities of grabbing, adversities of no apparent concern to this child.

In the following dialogue, after training, it is clear that the adult is now assuming a new role vis-á-vis the child. (Same type of problem, this time a mother):

> M: Ralph, what happened? What's the matter?
> C: He's got my racing car. He won't give it back.
> M: Why do you have to have it back now?
> C: Cause he's had a long turn.

In eliciting Ralph's point of view, this mother just learned something that would not have been possible had she simply demanded he share. She learned that, in fact, her son had shared his toy and that the problem to be solved was different than it first appeared to be: It was not merely a matter of wanting the toy back; the second child had kept his toy for a "long turn." Further dialogue demonstrates the ICPS approach toward solution of the problem:

> M: How do you think your friend feels when you grab toys?
> C: Mad, but I don't care. It's mine.
> M: What did your friend do when you grabbed the toy?
> C: He hit me but I want my toy.
> M: How did that make *you* feel?
> C: Mad.
> M: You're mad and your friend is mad, and he hit you. Can you think of a different way to get your toy back so you both won't be mad and so he won't hit you? (Shure & Spivack, 1978, pp. 36–37)

What Ralph would say at this point is not critical. What is critical is that Ralph is guided to think about the problem and what happened when he acted as he did. This mother focused on the child's view of the problem, wanting his toy back, and not what might have been her view, a need for her child to share or discontent with his having grabbed.

This is not to say adults should never show anger. Anger is a problem that a child has to learn to cope with. Nor should children always get what they want. They must learn to cope with frustration when they cannot have their wish. One child asked his teacher for some Play-Dough. She told him she could not get it now because she was tending to a child who was hurt. When asked if he could think of something different to do until she was finished, he thought for a minute, then said, "I'll go paint." Had the teacher suggested he paint, the child, no doubt, would have said "I don't want to paint, I want the Play-Dough." A child is much more likely to carry out *his/her own* idea than one suggested or demanded by an adult.

Research Findings

Within a wide IQ range (70–120+), teacher-trained nursery and kindergarten youngsters improved in both alternative solution and consequential thinking skills more than comparable nontrained controls. More importantly, trained children who most improved in these two skills were the same youngsters who most improved in behaviors characteristic of impulsivity and inhibition, supporting the theoretical position of ICPS skills as behavioral mediators. These thinking skills helped impulsive children learn to wait, become less overemotional when frustrated, less nagging and demanding, and less aggressive. Inhibited children became more socially outgoing, more able to stand up for their rights when attacked, and more expressive of their feelings. Of these two skills, however, it was the alternative solution thinking skills which emerged as the strongest behavioral mediator, and such was the case for both 4- and 5-year-olds. It appears that consequential thinking only guides a child's action if the child has a reasonable repertoire of solutions from which to choose. (For complete data and statistical analyses, see Shure & Spivack, 1980; Spivack & Shure, 1974)

One full year after training, there was no significant loss of ICPS skills. ICPS-trained children who began as impulsive or inhibited and were judged to be adjusted by their teachers immediately after training maintained that good adjustment when reevaluated by different teachers 1 and 2 years later. In addition, we learned that ICPS-trained children showing reasonably well adjusted behaviors in nursery school were likely to maintain those behaviors throughout kindergarten and first grade, more so than comparable nontrained controls. This finding is particularly important for primary prevention because it means that ICPS training helped to prevent the incidence of behavioral difficulties from occurring. (For detailed analyses, see Shure & Spivack, 1979; for evaluation measures, see Shure & Spivack, Notes 14 & 15).

The advantages of such programming become further evident when we note the percentage of adjusted, nontrained children steadily declining from the beginning of nursery to the end of the first grade. Such trends are further supported by the research of Spivack and Swift (1977), who demonstrated that behaviors in adjusted inner-city children regress still further by the end of the third grade, and by Zax and Cowen (1976), who report that more seriously disturbed youngsters, left untreated, are often quite impaired by the third grade. The ICPS approach, as measured through first grade, appears to show real promise as a technique to change this course.

In training mothers, it became clear that many were themselves poor problem solvers at the start. We learned that effects on children were greater when both mother and child were taught how to think. Mothers who developed skills to think through hypothetical mother-child or child-child problems; who could foresee potential obstacles; who could appreciate their child's point of view, even when different from their own; and who could recognize that the child needed to think independently about problem solutions were also more likely to encourage their children to think when real problems came up. While these new skills of the mother had significant impact on her child's ICPS skills, it was still the child's resultant ICPS skills that had the most significant, direct impact on his behavior. We assert that as children are freed to think for themselves and acquire skills to do that, impulsive children have less need to be impatient or aggressive; the inhibited, less need to withdraw from people and from problems they cannot solve. When not told what or what not to do everytime a problem comes up, children can generalize these skills to better deal with problematic situations. This became particularly evident when children trained by their mothers at home significantly improved on a number of school behavioral dimensions as measured by teachers. (Complete data and parent measures are detailed in Shure & Spivack, 1978; Shure, 1979; in press a, b.)

What is it about the training that produces ability to generalize newly acquired skills? We believe it has to do with the ability to think for oneself. Instead of teaching adult-valued "good" ways to solve problems, young children were taught to consider alternatives and the consequences. The goal was not immediate resolution of the problem. It was more important to help the child recognize the problem, what might have led up to it, and to consider the various solutions available. Encouraging children to think like this would, in our view, add to their understanding of what to do in real-life interpersonal situations.

Evaluation

The evaluation of interventions for use by teachers and/or parents must consider both practical program and scientific research considerations. Without considering practical subtleties of implementation, training agents can misuse or misinterpret the critical features of what the intervention is supposed to convey. Without appreciating the finer points of research methodology and interpretation of outcome, erroneous conclusions about program impact can result. It is the consideration of both that gives a program the potential for wider applicability and effective utilization.

Program Considerations

Any intervention is only as effective as the agent who conducts it. No matter how enthusiastic a teacher may be to implement the ICPS program, it soon became clear that teachers of older children often require more orientation toward the program's focus than teachers of younger children. Our research has shown that fifth grade teachers sometimes need more training to focus on interpersonal conflicts as problems to be solved, rather than simply as annoyances or disturbances to be dealt with quickly and be rid of. Perhaps teachers of younger children are from the start more oriented toward helping children adapt behaviorally to school, whereas teachers of older children are more oriented toward curriculum. As one fifth-grade teacher commented, "Before training, when minor problems came up, I just gave them the eye, they knew what I meant, and they sat down and forgot about it. Now I ask them to think of a way to solve it, and they usually can." As another teacher said, "I learned that what might seem little to me is not always little to the child."

In addition to basic orientation toward the general approach, a central element of ICPS intervention is the use of earlier described problem-solving communications or dialogues. Twenty to 40 minutes of structured formal lessons, even if conducted four or five times a week over a 3- to 4-month period, is not enough. Teachers and parents must continue to use such dialogues in actual problem situations for the positive effects to be reinforced. Interventions that include application of ICPS skills to real problems through the use of dialogues obtain significantly greater behavioral changes (e.g., Allen, 1978; Wowkanech, Note 7) than those that do not (e.g., Sharp, Note 16; Durlack & Sherman, Note 17).

A further note on dialoguing: We learned early on that logistics of implementation by fifth-grade teachers would be considerably more difficult than by teachers of the younger children. Unlike teachers of nursery and kindergarten youngsters who supervised the children both indoors and out, teachers of fifth-graders were seldom outside on the playground at recess or participating during the lunch hour. Any dialoguing that took place generally occurred only in the classroom itself. Because of this, fifth-grade teachers were often not likely to dialogue on-the-spot with those involved in the conflict. When dialogues did occur in the classroom, frequently teachers involved the whole class. The whole-group technique can be very effective, except that it does not give the youngster who has the problem a chance to put his/her ideas into effect. One way to overcome the large group obstacle is, at the suggestion of one of our more creative teachers, to have children role-play (act out) actual problems, and if they happened in the classroom, to do so as soon after they occurred as possible. Since role-playing was part of the formal script for contrived problems, the children were able to learn from this experience, often quite successfully. In time, most of our teachers did learn to dialogue and to take advantage of opportunities to talk with specific children.

Research Considerations: Methodology

One inherent difficulty of evaluation of teacher-as-agent ICPS intervention from a research perspective arises when teachers who conduct the training also assess behavior change. The ideal design would be to create a situation wherein children are taken out of the classroom by independent staff, some receiving the training and some not. The teacher, unaware of child group placement, could then objectively rate each child's behavior prior to and following training, completely free of bias and ego involvement. The problem with this design is that if the teachers are not involved in the training, they do not know which children to engage in dialogue. One way to circumvent this obstacle is for the teachers to do the training, but have independent outside observers judge the children's behavior before and after intervention. This is also difficult because an observer, by spending enough time with the children, would soon learn that some children were being treated uniquely in the classroom.

Peer ratings, another procedure to overcome rater bias, is also problematic. While peer and teacher behavior ratings correlate well before training, our inner-city fifth-grade children were less able to perceive changes in behavior when compared to the teacher sample (Shure, Note 18). As this may well have been a function of the particular peer rating scale used in that study, further testing is being conducted. Perhaps the most reliable and cost-effective independent ratings could come from other teachers whose classes children attend. By fifth grade, most schools provide classes taught by various specialty teachers. Their ratings could be compiled and analyzed.

Although our future research with older elementary school children will add independent ratings by outside observers, our evaluations of impact on preschoolers, kindergartens, and fifth-graders have thus far been based on different research control strategies. First, teachers rated several behavioral items in addition to those of research training concern. This procedure tested for overall "halo effects" of behavioral improvement. In all studies to date, no such halo occurred. Therefore, teachers did clearly discriminate ICPS relevant and nonrelevant items. Second, our ICPS behavior change relationship analyses further highlighted teacher objectivity. Those ICPS skills that most strongly related to adjustment measures before training also showed the strongest relationship after training, especially alternative solution thinking skills.

In order to further test teacher-rating objectivity and the validity of ICPS behavioral impact, follow-up studies were conducted. At 6 month follow-up, kindergarten teachers rated the nursery youngsters remarkably similar to ratings of the nursery teachers at the end of the training period. Nursery trained youngsters not receiving the second (kindergarten) year of ICPS exposure continued to be rated similarly by different teachers throughout the first grade. Thus, children judged by their nursery teachers to have improved in their behavior were judged as displaying adjusted, adaptive behaviors by later teachers who were completely unaware of the training or the child's earlier experiences with it.

Perhaps still more convincing were our findings for children trained by their mothers at home and rated by their teachers in school. Those teachers were not only unaware of the child's ICPS scores, but were also unaware of which children were trained and the child's training performance. If lack of independent raters in our nursery training research created a suspicion of teacher-rater bias, ratings by our follow-up kindergarten teachers and teachers of our mother-trained children clearly allayed that doubt.

A further, though related, methodological issue concerns how much the training agent is told about the program goals during the research stage. Our research training teachers and mothers were told of the cognitive problem-solving goals but not the behavioral goals in an attempt to keep their behavior ratings objective. In contrast, teachers (nursery only) who were later given ICPS training in a purely service capacity were, unlike the research teachers, told of both the cognitive and behavioral goals. Telling about both was judged reasonable for two reasons: (1) to interest a wider range of teachers and (2) the research theory testing stage was completed. Importantly, the ratings by service teachers of children's behavioral improvement showed percentages remarkably similar to those in the research years. This finding suggests that even if the research teachers had learned of the behavioral goals, the results would likely not have been different from those obtained. (For further discussion of these issues see Shure, 1979.)

Finally, though there are no doubt many other methodological considerations for evaluating the validity of any intervention, we also considered the placebo issue. In one study (Shure, Spivack, & Gordon, 1972), a placebo group was included in which small groups of children engaged in finger games, animal imitations, and other nonproblem-solving activities—activities which were, as those of the ICPS training groups, designed to stimulate mutual teacher-child interaction. This study, a pilot, was conducted outside of the classroom by the senior author and research staff for the purpose of obtaining first hand reactions of the children included and not included in the program. Thus, as in the Sharp (Note 16) and Durlack (Note 17) studies, children were taken from the classroom, preventing any dialoguing techniques to be extended into actual classroom problems during the day. While these research staff ICPS-trained groups did not show behavior change as dramatic as teacher ICPS-trained groups, they did show significantly greater improvement than either the placebo or an included no-treatment control.

It might also be asked whether small group teacher-child interaction alone might produce greater posttest performance and/or behavioral improvement. In our research, all no-treatment control classes had such small group interactions (e.g., reading groups, story time), thereby constituting natural built-in placebo groups. In all cases, ICPS-trained groups exceeded formal research placebos as well as natural built-in ones. Having discovered all this, our decision not to include formal research placebo groups in our large scale teacher-training research was a practical rather than a theoretical one. Given the natural placebos already existing in the classroom, it was judged more fruitful to test the impact of ICPS intervention on as many children and as many different teachers as staff time and existing work force would allow.

Not only did ICPS intervention groups fare better than placebo groups, but they also fared better than another intervention technique designed to improve classroom behavior. Wowkanech compared an ICPS-trained group with a modeling group. ICPS-trained children were more likely to generate their own solutions during actual conflict and to turn to different ones when needed. In contrast, the modeling group was more limited in the solutions they could generate. They more often resorted to hitting, grabbing, and other behaviors characteristic of impulsivity. If unsuccessful, these children more likely gave up in frustration or with a sense of failure.

Research Considerations: Impact

In addition to nursery and kindergarten aged children, ICPS intervention can be applied with other age groups as well. Elardo and Caldwell (1979) found the impulsive and prosocial behaviors of fourth and fifth graders can be improved by ICPS training (Elardo & Cooper, 1977). However, such improvement occurred only when the program was implemented for the entire school year and when all staff, not just teachers, consistently applied informal dialogues for real problems. This suggests the possibility that for success with older children, it is optimal to create a total problem-solving atmosphere within the school setting. This, if feasible, is one option. A more practical school option for this age group entails relying upon a single training agent (i.e., the teacher), but we found that in a 3- to 4-month training period, use of single ICPS training agents did not have as dramatic an impact on maladaptive behaviors as on positive prosocial ones (Shure, Note 18). It simply may take longer for a single training agent to change maladaptive behaviors, not an illogical possibility. Weissberg and his colleagues (Notes 9 & 19), who also used single-agent trainers (teachers) similarly, reported only some immediate behavior change in third graders.

Program difficulties with older children notwithstanding, Gesten and others (Note 20) report that a year later, the Weissberg-trained study children were less likely than controls to show further behavior problems. This has special significance for primary prevention, as such intervention reversed the natural tendency, as previously described by Spivack and Swift (1977) and Zax and Cowen (1976), for increased behavior problems as children get older.

We conclude that if educators and clinicians have assumed that believing emotional tension paves the way for one to think straight, research reported here supports the reverse idea, that ability to think straight can pave the way for emotional relief. While we make no claim that ICPS training is the single best means to achieving primary prevention, we believe that behavior is guided more by how people think than by what they think. We also believe that the quality of social adjustment and interpersonal competence can be noticeably enhanced, and later maladaption dramatically reduced, by implementing the problem-solving approach to adjustment.

REFERENCE NOTES

    1.   Spivack, G., Standen, C., Bryson, J., & Garrett, L. *Interpersonal problem-solving thinking among the elderly.* Paper presented at the meeting of the American Psychological Association, Toronto, August 1978.
    2.   Shure, M. B., & Spivack, G. *A preventive mental health program for four-year-old Head Start children.* Paper presented at the meeting of the Society for Research in Child Development, Philadelphia, March 1973.
    3.   Pellegrini, D. Social cognition, competence, and adaptation in children under stress. In N. Garmezy (Chair), *Studies of stress and coping in children.* Symposium presented at the meeting of the American Psychological Association, Montreal, September 1980.
    4.   Coché, E. *Therapeutic benefits of a problem-solving training program for hospitalized psychiatric patients.* Paper presented at the meeting of the Society of Psychotherapy Research, San Diego, 1976.

5. Spivack, G., & Levine, M. *Self-regulation in acting-out and normal adolescents* (Report M-4531). Washington, D.C.: National Institute of Health, 1973.
6. Appel, P. W., Kaestner, E., & Sofer, S. Personal communication, 1975.
7. Wowkanech, N. Personal communication, August 26, 1978.
8. Camp, B. W., & Bash, M. A. *The classroom "Think Aloud" program.* Paper presented at the meeting of the American Psychological Association, Toronto, August 1978.
9. Weissberg, R., Gesten, E., Rapkin, B., Boike, M., Cowen, E., Davidson, E., Flores de Apodaca, R., McKim, B., & Rains, M. *Interpersonal problem-solving training: A competence building program for children.* Paper presented at the American Psychological Association, New York, September 1979.
10. Nesbitt-Brown, A. Personal communication, June 16, 1978.
11. Platt, J. J., Morell, J., & Flaherty, E. Personal communication, July 2, 1980.
12. Shure, M. B., & Spivack, G. *Solving interpersonal problems: A program for four-year-old nursery school children: Training script.* Philadelphia: Hahnemann Medical College, Department of Mental Health Sciences, 1971.
13. Shure, M. B., & Spivack, G. *A mental health program for kindergarten children: Training script.* Philadelphia: Hahnemann Medical College, Department of Mental Health Sciences, 1974. (a)
14. Shure, M. B., & Spivack, G. *Preschool interpersonal problemsolving (PIPS) test: Manual.* Philadelphia: Hahnemann Medical College, Department of Mental Health Sciences, 1974. (b)
15. Shure, M. B., & Spivack, G. *A mental health program for preschool and kindergarten children, and a mental health program for mothers of young children: An interpersonal problem-solving approach toward social adjustment. A comprehensive report of research and training* (No. MH-20372). Washington, D.C.: National Institute of Mental Health, 1975.
16. Sharp, K. *Impact of interpersonal problem-solving training on preschoolers' behavioral adjustment.* Paper presented at the meeting of the American Psychological Association, New York, September 1979.
17. Durlak, J. A., & Sherman, D. Primary prevention of school maladjustment. In J. A. Durlak (Chair), *Behavioral approaches to primary prevention: Programs, outcomes, and issues.* Symposium presented at the meeting of the American Psychological Association, New York, September 1979.
18. Shure, M. B. *Interpersonal problem-solving in ten-year-olds* (Final Report No. MH-27741). Washington, D.C.: National Institute of Mental Health, 1980.
19. Weissberg, R. P., Gesten, E. L., Liebenstein, N. L., Schmid, K. D., & Hutton, H. *The Rochester social problem-solving (SPS) program: A training manual for teachers of 2nd–4th grade children.* Rochester, NY: Center for Community Study, 1979.
20. Gesten, E. L., Weissberg, R. P., Rapkin, B., Davidson, E., & Bowen, G. *Effects of a third grade social problem-solving training program: A one-year follow up.* In preparation.

REFERENCES

Allen, G., Chinsky, J., Larcen, S., Lochman, J., & Selinger, H. *Community psychology and the schools: A behaviorally oriented multilevel preventive approach.* Hillsdale, NJ: Earlbaum, 1976.
Allen, R. J. *An investigatory study of the effects of a cognitive approach to interpersonal problem-solving on the behavior of emotionally upset psychosocially deprived preschool children.* Unpublished doctoral dissertation, Center for Minority Studies, Brookings Institute, Union Graduate School, Washington, D.C., 1978.

Bensky, J. M. *Differential effectiveness of a social problem solving curriculum with regular and special education children.* Unpublished doctoral dissertation, University of Connecticut, Storrs, 1978.

Elardo, P. T., & Caldwell, B. M. The effects of an experimental social development program on children in the middle childhood period. *Psychology in the Schools,* 1979, *16*, 93–100.

Elardo, P. T., & Cooper, M. *Aware: Activities for social development.* Menlo Park, CA: Addison-Wesley, 1977.

Elias, M. J. *The development of a theory-based measure of how children understand and attempt to resolve problematic social situations.* Unpublished masters thesis, University of Connecticut, Storrs, 1978.

Enright, R. D. An integration of social cognitive development and cognitive processing: Educational applications. *American Educational Research Journal,* 1980, *17*, 21–41.

Gotlib, I., & Asarnow, R. F. Interpersonal and impersonal problem-solving skills in mildly clinically depressed university students. *Journal of Consulting and Clinical Psychology,* 1979, *47*, 86–95.

Healey, K. *An investigation of the relationship between certain social cognitive abilities and social behavior, and the efficacy of training in social cognitive skills for elementary retarded educable children.* Unpublished doctoral dissertation, Bryn Mawr College, 1977.

Intagliata, J. Increasing the interpersonal problem-solving skills of an alcoholic population. *Journal of Consulting and Clinical Psychology,* 1978, *46*, 489–498.

McClure, L. F., Chinsky, J. M., & Larcen, S. W. Enhancing social problem-solving performance in an elementary school setting. *Journal of Educational Psychology,* 1978, *70*, 504–513.

Platt, J. J., & Spivack, G. Studies in problem-solving thinking of psychiatric patients: Patient-control differences and factorial structure of problem-solving thinking. *Proceedings of the 81st Annual Convention of the American Psychological Association,* 1973, *8*, 461–462. (Summary)

Platt, J. J., Spivack, G., Altman, N., Altman, D., & Peizer, S. B. Adolescent problem-solving thinking. *Journal of Consulting and Clinical Psychology,* 1974, *42*, 787–793.

Shure, M. B. Training children to solve interpersonal problems: A preventive mental health program. In R. E. Muñoz, L. R. Snowden, & J. G. Kelly (Eds.), *Social and psychological research in community settings.* San Francisco: Jossey-Bass, 1979.

Shure, M. B. Social competence as a problem-solving skill. In J. Wine & M. Smye (Eds.), *Social competence.* New York: Guilford Press, in press. (a)

Shure, M. B. Interpersonal problem-solving: A cog in the wheel of social cognition. In F. C. Serafica (Ed.), *Social cognition, context, and social behavior: A developmental perspective.* New York: Guilford Press, in press. (b)

Shure, M. B., & Spivack, G. Means-ends thinking, adjustment and social class among elementary school-aged children. *Journal of Consulting and Clinical Psychology,* 1972, *38*, 348–353.

Shure, M. B., & Spivack, G. *Problem-solving techniques in childrearing.* San Francisco: Jossey-Bass, 1978.

Shure, M. B., & Spivack, G. Interpersonal cognitive problem-solving and primary prevention: Programming for preschool and kindergarten children. *Journal of Clinical Child Psychology,* 1979, *2*, 89–94.

Shure, M. B., & Spivack, G. Interpersonal problem-solving as a mediator of behavioral adjustment in preschool and kindergarten children. *Journal of Applied Developmental Psychology,* 1980, *1*, 29–43.

Shure, M. B., Spivack, G., & Gordon, R. Problem-solving thinking: A preventive mental health program for preschool children. *Reading World,* 1972, *11*, 259–273.

Spivack, G. Problem-solving thinking and mental health. *The Forum*, 1973, 2, 58–73.
Spivack, G., Platt, J. J., & Shure, M. B. *The problem-solving approach to adjustment*. San Francisco: Jossey-Bass, 1976.
Spivack, G., & Shure, M. B. *Social adjustment of young children*. San Francisco: Jossey-Bass, 1974.
Spivack, G., & Swift, M. "High risk" classroom behaviors in kindergarten and first grade. *American Journal of Community Psychology*, 1977, 5, 385–397.
Steinlauf, B. Problem-solving skills, locus of control, and the contraceptive effectiveness of young women. *Child Development*, 1979, 50, 268–271.
Zax, M., & Cowen, E. L. *Abnormal psychology: Changing conceptions* (2nd ed.). New York: Holt, Rinehart and Winston, 1976.

EVALUATION OF PROGRAMS SEEKING TO ASSIST ADULT LEARNERS IN HOME, SCHOOL, AND CAREER TRANSITIONS

Ronald H. Miller

ABSTRACT. The 1970s brought many information and counseling service programs into existence to assist adult learners in home, school, and career transitions. However, the evaluations of these programs to date generally have been one-shot case studies. A nonequivalent control group quasi-experimental design was utilized to evaluate the information program of an urban information and referral center for adult learners. Results of the evaluation indicated that the information program was effective in contrast with no treatment and that the original assumptions in program planning were imprecise. Such evaluation designs are required to answer more sophisticated questions on justification, improvement, and planning of adult learning programs. Evaluations are needed to explain participation, persistence, and satisfaction in adult learning programs; to explicate effectiveness as a function of program development assumptions; and to monitor program progress on local, state, and national levels in meeting societal needs. Considerable physiological and emotional stress may result from transitions experienced by adults, and lifelong learning programs may play an important role in preventing or ameliorating that stress.

Programs to serve the needs of adults seeking to make home, school, and career transitions proliferated in the late 1970s and are likely to flourish in the 1980s as a result of the demand for such services. A national survey of adult career counseling needs conducted by the College Entrance Examination Board (Arbeiter, Aslanian, Schmerbeck, & Brickell, 1978a) found that nearly 40 million Americans were or anticipated being in a state of career transition. Programs have been developed on college campuses (for example, women's centers), as well as in the community (for

Reprints may be obtained from Ronald H. Miller, Assistant Director, Professional Studies, Continuing Education Program, Queens College, 65-30 Kissena Boulevard, Flushing, NY 11367. I am most grateful to Lawrence B. Mohr, the University of Michigan, and Marilyn D. Jacobson, Northwestern University, for comments to earlier versions of this article.

Prevention in Human Services, Vol. 1(1/2), Fall/Winter 1981

example, educational brokering agencies). Jacobson (Note 1) indicated that more than 350 organizations in the country currently conduct programs which:

1. attempt to provide accurate, current labor market information which includes the tasks, skills, and credentials associated with jobs,
2. interpret information by use of evaluation and comparison criteria,
3. examine attitudes, interests, and values of people, and
4. provide information regarding education and training.

These programs frequently deal with a very real problem—the human needs of people unemployed or who anticipate a career change which might include some period of unemployment. According to Taber, Walsh, and Cooke (1979):

> Previous research on unemployment has shown that people whose employment is suddenly terminated, or who anticipate such termination, show physiological signs of strain such as elevated blood pressure (related to heart disease and hypertension) elevated uric acid (related to gout), and elevated pulse rate (related to feelings of tension) .... Such individuals may also display psychological strains such as depressed mood, diminished self-esteem, and lowered satisfaction with life. Additionally, their family relationships may become severely strained. (p. 134)

Services for adults in transition may prevent some of the physiological and emotional stresses of life. They are one of many social services necessary for a productive and healthy citizenry. There are circumstances in some communities where a major plant or industry has shut down and an entire community linked these transition services with the work of local social service agencies. A good illustration is Mansfield, Ohio, where substantial retraining and reemployment of a workforce previously in the tire and rubber industry has been achieved (Abbott, Note 2).

The common denominator in all programs which seek to assist adult learners in home, school, and career transitions is some form of information and counseling service. These services are needed to link clients with potential learning resources (Cross, 1978).

Program Evaluation

Grotelueschen (1980) has analyzed evaluation efforts in the area of adult learning and suggests that there are three purposes which may be involved in such evaluation: program justification (past oriented), program improvement (present oriented),and program planning (future oriented). In addition, programs should be examined from four perspectives: goals, designs, implementations, and outcomes. Finally, program components such as participants, instructors, topics, and contexts should be assessed with respect to the perspectives of the program.

Evaluation of programs seeking to assist adult learners in home, school, and career transitions is in its infancy. Currently, there are few summative evaluation reports with conclusive results regarding the impact of participation in the learning activity on the learner's performance in family, work, and community (Knox, 1979). Studies of educational and career counseling services in libraries (Toombs & Croyle, Note 3; Toombs, Note 4), in a state administered external degree program (Dyer, Note 5), in a telephone counseling service for home-based adults (Arbeiter, et al., 1978b), in seven communities across the country (Paltridge, Regan, & Terkla, Note 6), and in a regional agency which links potential learners with learning resources (Kordalewski and Alamprese-Johnson, Note 7) deal with the impact of services on clients. These studies tend to be of the one-shot case study variety. There is some evidence that some treatment had some effect on a client. We generally cannot ascertain whether alternative treatments might have had a more marked impact or how different nonparticipants were from participants. Now that these programs have proliferated and initial program evaluation experience has been reported, evaluators of programs seeking to assist adult learners in home, school, and career transitions need to begin designing studies which can answer more sophisticated questions on justification, improvement, and planning of programs.

The following program evaluation of an information and referral center for adult learners in an urban area was developed from an actual situation and is presented to illustrate how more rigorous quasi-experimental evaluation designs can be utilized. Since many of these programs are often supported at least partially by federal, state, and local government funds (Christoffel, Ehrlich, & Macy, 1978) as well as by private foundations and client fees, program evaluation is becoming critical to service providers in developing long-range effectiveness and to policymakers and funding sources in making investment decisions.

Evaluation of Urban Information Center

With funding from a federal grant, the Urban Information Center (UIC) was created in 1972 to address the problem of urban adults' lack of information concerning local continuing education opportunities. The UIC was opened to the public in January 1974 after compiling information on the more than 550 units of 330 organizations offering postsecondary education for adults in a large city in the northeastern United States. Limited evaluation research on client satisfaction and service impact was undertaken through June 1974. With a new funding cycle starting in July 1974, the UIC director wanted better evaluation information for justification, improvement, and planning of the program.

An objective for program evaluation was established: No more than 266,000 persons in the city will lack information on continuing education opportunities during the period July 1, 1974 through June 30, 1975 (Deniston, Note 8). Conditions of the federal funding dictated that the target population be those adults seeking to continue their education at institutions offering instruction beyond high school (termed postsecondary education).

Tabulations of educational attainment provided by the census bureau for adults 25 years of age or older included 1,733,140 persons in 1970 in the prime postsecondary education audience (these are people with a high school degree or some college education). Utilizing the finding by the Commission on Non-Traditional Study (1973) indicating that 16.5% of the general adult population in the United States finds lack of knowledge of existing education opportunities a barrier to participation, project staff estimated 286,000 residents of the city each year would not continue their education due to a lack of information about existing educational opportunities. The constant influx of immigrants plus the probable census bureau undercount of minority group populations in the city made program staff feel that the 286,000 persons annually needing assistance represented a conservative estimate of the problem magnitude and that this figure would remain constant each year during the next decade.

A planned attainment rate for the UIC was established for the period July 1, 1974 through June 30, 1975. Planned attainment can be represented by the expression $(G - P)/G$ where G is the number of persons residing in the city who are in the previously mentioned target audience who lack information about existing continuing education opportunities and P is planned attainment (in this case the number of persons who lack information on continuing education opportunities at the end of the funding year). The UIC director assumed that 20,000 people was a reasonable number of clients for the program to serve in one year. Thus, the attainment rate can be expressed as: $(286,000 - 266,000)/286,000 = 7.0\%$. For the forthcoming year, the UIC director set a subobjective that 500,000 city residents in the target audience of the program know about the educational information service of the UIC (Deniston, Note 9).

The UIC director in consultation with the advisory board and the funding agency planned the following activities for July 1, 1974 through June 30, 1975:

1. Continuing education opportunities in the 550 units of the 330 organizations offering instruction will be recorded and organized for staff use continuously during the year.
2. People will be given information on continuing education opportunities on the telephone, through the mail, and in person.
3. City residents will be informed of the availability of the service of the UIC through public service advertising in the subways, advertising in 20 local newspapers and magazines, posters displayed in 200 library branches, public service announcements on local radio stations, and by referrals from education and community organizations.

Design of Evaluation

The UIC's experimental program was an information and referral service on continuing education programs in a major metropolitan area. The program maintained files on approximately 20,000 courses and programs for the 1974–75 academic year.

The experimental group in the evaluation of UIC was made up of those clients who contacted the referral service. Most often, contact was made by telephone, through the use of a widely publicized telephone number. Some mail requests for information were also received, and a relatively small number of walk-in clients were also serviced. Three distinct outreach efforts were mounted; one in the fall, one in the winter, and one in the spring.

The control group for the evaluation was constituted by drawing a random sample of residents in the area where the IUC program was operating. The sample was constructed to reflect the socioeconomic characteristics of the UIC service area. A further requirement for control group membership was that a person must not have contacted UIC.

The UIC program was evaluated using a nonequivalent control group design (Campbell & Stanley, 1966) with three replications. The initial evaluation was in Fall 1974, the second in Winter 1974–75, and the third in Spring/Summer 1975.

Data was collected from respondents concerning demographic variables and their needs for continuing education opportunities. Because of the more extensive contact which was possible with members of the experimental group, more detailed information was collected for those individuals. A summary of the information collected (and for which groups) appears in Table 1.

The crucial outcome variables were "known continuing education opportunity choices" and "educational attainment." The technique used to measure program effectiveness was analysis of covariance using estimated true scores as covariates. A detailed description of this approach is discussed in Porter and Chibucos (1974). The lack of true random assignment in this experiment made it necessary to employ imperfect correction factors for the estimation of true score means. Even with this limitation, analysis of covariance is the most powerful statistical analysis that is available for this situation.

Utilization rates were also seasonally adjusted before statistical analysis was performed. This was necessary because of traditional fluctuations which take place in the demand for postsecondary education services. The highest demand rate is in the fall, followed by winter and spring/summer. Based on our experience with these fluctuations, respective weights of .5, .4, and .1 were employed. (A detailed technical description of data collection and analysis can be obtained by writing to the author.)

There are several reasons why this design was applied in the evaluation of the UIC:

1. Clients of the program are members of the city population who have selected themselves for treatment by contacting the organization. No control group is available for this same population of clients. Thus, construction of a control group is required to evaluate the treatment.

Table 1

Information Obtained From Control

And Experimental Groups

Item	Control Groups	Experimental Groups
Age	X	X
Educational attainment	X	X
Ethnic background	X	X
Family (or individual) income	X	X
How person discovered known sources of information	X	X
How person discovered the program		X
Helpfulness of the program		X
Known continuing education opportunity choices	X	X
Marital status	X	X
Number of institutions contacted as a result of information supplied by the program		X
Occupation	X	X
Reasons for wanting to take advantage of continuing education opportunities	X	X
Sex	X	X
Sources of information used in locating continuing education opportunities	X	X
Subject interested in taking	X	X
Suggestions for program improvement		X

2. Data provided by the control, regardless of its manner of selection, assists in the appropriate analysis of the null hypothesis—information on continuing education opportunity choices an individual has.

3. Confidence in the interpretation of evaluation results is enhanced by the threats to internal validity which are controlled by utilization of this design—history, maturation, testing, instrumentation, selection, and mortality (Campbell & Stanley, 1966).

This design, however, does not rule out the possibilities of regression effects and interaction of selection and maturation. (External threats to validity also are not ruled out.) Yet, despite these problems, the design allows information to be gained relating to the null hypothesis which otherwise would not be obtained.

Results

Data collected in the evaluation process yielded the following conclusions:

1. An important objective of the program was that no more than 266,000 persons in the city would lack information on continuing education opportunities during the period July 1, 1974 through June 30, 1975. Results in Table 1 indicate that project staff had used the wrong figure for estimating the total number of persons in the target audience with no information on continuing education opportunities prior to the beginning of the program. The results indicate that G is 256,311 rather than the 286,000, which was the initial assumption.

According to program records, 6,300 clients in the target audience used the service during the year in question. Another 4,200 persons not in the target audience also used the service. (This suggests an expanded definition of the target audience.) The attainment rate can be represented by the expression $(G - A)/G$ where G is the state of the world and A is the actual attainment. Using information gained from this study, the actual attainment equation yields the following result: $(256,331 - 250,031)/256,311 = 2.5\%$. Therefore, the UIC did not meet its planned attainment rate of 7.0%. However, the result is sensitive to the definition of the target audience, and a different definition which might better fit the entire population served by the program would produce a more meaningful result in favor of the treatment.

2. Comparisons between experimental and control groups were made by the use of covariance analysis using correction factors for the effects of nonrandom assignment. The dependent variable for these analyses was "knowledge of continuing education opportunities." Within each control-experimental comparison, two separate analyses were performed; one for people with 1 to 3 years of college and one for those with up to 4 years of high school. (These two classifications defined the target audiences as mandated by the funding agency). In four of the six comparisons, the information treatment produced higher knowledge scores in the

Table 2

Estimated Number of People Lacking Information

on Continuing Education Opportunities

Group	Number with no information	Percent of sample	Baseline figure	Weighting	Estimated total
E 1	200	23.5	1,733,140	0.5	203,644
E 2	125	20.8	1,733,140	0.4	144,197
E 3	50	7.7	1,733,140	0.1	13,345
Subtotal	375	17.9	1,733,140	0.5	180,593
C 1	50	6.3	1,733,140	0.5	54,594
C 2	100	11.1	1,733,140	0.4	76,951
C 3	75	11.5	1,733,140	0.1	19,931
Subtotal	225	9.6	1,733,140	0.5	75,738
Total	600	13,5	1,733,140	1.0	256,331

E 1,2,3 : Experimental groups (August 15-October 15, 1974; December 15, 1974-February 15, 1975; April 15, 1975-June 15, 1975).

C 1,2,3 : Control groups (August 15-October 15, 1974; December 15, 1974-February 15, 1975; April 15, 1975-June 15, 1975).

experimental group than in the control group. This pattern was reversed in two of the six cases.

We believe the obtained results are reasonable in light of the fact that a large amount of information on continuing education was distributed by the experimental program and that the program was operating in an area where many people already had considerable knowledge of continuing education opportunities. Therefore, the information treatment generally was effective in contrast with no treatment.

An analysis of covariance test for interaction between the treatment groups and educational attainment indicated there was no significant interaction effect. This finding adds strength to the finding that the information treatment was effective.

3. While the UIC did not attain its subobjective (500,000 city residents in the program's target audience knowing about the educational information service of the UIC), it did communicate to a substantial population in the metropolitan region. A different definition of target audience might have lead to attainment of the subobjective. The figures developed in Table 4 do not include persons who knew about the service but who were not in the target audience. So, in all likelihood, it appears that the program was known to more than 500,000 city residents.

Discussion

The use of powerful evaluation strategies in adult education programs is important for three reasons: program monitoring, knowledge of how participants relate to programs, and understanding of program effectiveness as it relates to program implementation and development activities.

Table 3

Mean Difference in Knowledge of
Continuing Education Opportunities

Treatment groups compared	Education attainment	Corrected pretest difference	Posttest difference	F
E$_1$,C$_1$	4 yrs HS	-1.1	-0.3	87.5*
	1-3 yrs Col	-0.7	-0.1	180.9*
E$_2$,C$_2$	4 yrs HS	0.0	-0.9	58.5*
	1-3 yrs Col	-0.2	0.1	20.7*
E$_3$,C$_3$	4 yrs HS	0.0	2.3	64.8*
	1-3 yrs Col	-1.0	-1.3	103.3*

* $p < .001$

Table 4

Estimated Number of People
With Knowledge of UIC

Group	Number with no information	Percent of sample	Baseline figure	Weighting	Estimated total
C 1	200	25.0	1,733,140	0.5	216,643
C 2	240	26.7	1,733,140	0.4	185,099
C 3	130	20.0	1,733,140	0.1	34,663
Total	570	24.3	1,733,140	1.0	436,405

Monitoring

Society has a considerable stake in the success of adult learning programs, and that stake is reflected in oversight responsibilities at the local, state, and federal levels. According to the Future Directions for a Learning Society program of the College Board, in the next 20 years (Glover & Gross, 1979):

1. Help is needed for workers whose skills are in low demand to make mid-career transitions.
2. Lifelong learning opportunities must be geared to available career opportunities as well as individual needs and aspirations.
3. Functional literacy for the disadvantaged to reduce social dependence and unequal educational and employment opportunities is required.
4. The aged will need help in preparing for successful retirement, which will include satisfactory part-time employment.

Given these needs for lifelong learning, oversight bodies and funding agencies must have information on whether continuing education programs for adults are functioning efficiently and effectively. The UIC attainment record on its subobjective for 1974–75 was unusual since similar operations do not seek out large numbers of potential adult learners (Gould & Cross, 1972). On the basis of its 1974–75 record, the UIC was given additional grant support.

Participants in Programs

Evaluation studies can be used to explain participation, persistence, and satisfaction in adult learning programs. We would not only gain insights on how to achieve equal access to educational opportunities, but would also gain new knowledge on the elements of program design that facilitate adult learning. Currently, researchers are far short of adequate concepts and theories to explain adult participation. The evidence is clear that important segments of our society are underrepresented in organized learning activities for adults: blacks, people with less than a high school education, people with family incomes under $8,000, people aged 45 or older, and people living in central cities and on farms. Careful evaluation studies are needed to determine how programs might increase the participation of these groups in continuing education programs.

Effectiveness as a Function of Program Implementation and Development

Traditionally, adult learning programs have been developed and implemented on the basis of two major concepts: barriers and transitions. If barriers to participation are not ameliorated, learning activities will not be undertaken. Barriers are three in number: situational, dispositional, and institutional (Cross & Zusman, Note 10). The situational barriers usually require an individual adult to modify personal status to allow for the addition of an educational activity. Personal time patterns must be changed, finances must be reallocated, child care frequently needs to be arranged, and transportation patterns must be altered (Houle, 1972). Dispositional barriers often relate to the needs of adults to learn for the sake of career and family considerations. Adults who have not had formal instruction in many years are often afraid they will fail. Yet, when they discover that they can succeed, adult learners are the best students. Institutional barriers are practices by educational providers which inhibit adults from access to learning opportunities. In recent years, institutions have changed scheduling patterns, fee structures, program offerings, support service availability, and moved more offerings into the community to facilitate greater adult enrollment.

The Commission on Non-Traditional Study (1973), in pointing out that lack of information on educational opportunities was a barrier to adult participation in education, also noted financial, time, and adult responsibility obstacles which were more significant in its national survey. An earlier national study (Johnstone & Rivera, 1965) discovered that public awareness of educational opportunities varied greatly by type of subject matter wanted; that information on these opportunities was unequally distributed throughout the adult population; and that when the same instructional offerings were provided in different institutional settings, they came to the attention of quite different groups in the population.

When examined in light of these findings, the UIC evaluation leaves many unanswered questions. The use of a second treatment, such as career counseling, would have provided the UIC with better information on each service and on planning assumptions. As examples of important issues which the evaluation did not resolve, consider the following: What difference in program effectiveness will result from programs designed around different clusters of barriers? How efficient is it for a program to attempt to deal with any particular combination of barriers? What is the cost-effectiveness of each unit of resources per combination of barriers?

The transitions concept has emerged from adult development theory. There seem to be several major life cycle stages which most people have, for example, getting married, the birth of children, the last child entering school, and retirement. Life events provide the opportunity for personal growth (or deterioration.) Schlossberg (Note 11) suggests that to study adults in transition, one must look at characteristics of the particular transition, of the individual, and of environments of the adult both before and after the transition. Aslanian and Brickell (1980) found that the overwhelming reason why adults sought some type of learning was a life transition. The life areas in which these transitions occur are career, family, health, religion, citizenship, art, and leisure. Of the 83% who cited a life transition as causing them to seek learning, 92% were triggered by career or family events. According to the Aslanian and Brickell study, adults enter a learning experience in one status and expect to leave it in another.

The study of career transitions and appropriate information and guidance services suggested that personality characteristics and occupational status or classification should be studied for its impact on service needs (Arbeiter et al., 1978a). If a life event indeed triggers an adult to learn, the success of the transition may depend upon the success of the learning. Evaluation studies can be designed to test this assumption and to suggest improvements for programs which use the transition concept as a basic principle of program design.

Increasingly, programs for adult learners are attempting to combine barrier and transition concepts in order to develop powerful and successful programs. Are those combinations effective, however, and if not, how can they be improved? These are precisely the types of questions that can be answered with powerful evaluation designs.

The need for continuing education is often associated with a transition period in a person's life, and job, family, health, and age are all factors which may precipitate a stressful transition. In many cases, the availability of appropriate educational programs may play an important part in determining how quickly that transition is made and with what difficulty it takes place. With no knowledge of opportunities, no choice of appropriate instruction is possible. Lack of choice probably will lead to no consumption of education. While personal consumption of education does not always lead to the formation of human capital (which might, for example, assist in increasing lifetime earnings), often it does. Lack of human capital formation makes each person a less productive and less aware citizen. Society suffers from these deficiencies and as a result has to provide more public services (examples are welfare and unemployment insurance). With better evaluations of adult learning programs, a more proficient citizenry with less costs to society is attainable.

REFERENCE NOTES

1.   Jacobson, M. D. *Adult career advocates training program: Interim report.* Evanston, IL: Northwestern University School of Education, January 1979.
2.   Abbott, W. L. *The Mansfield formula for worker renewal.* Washington, D.C.: Service Center for Community and College Labor Union Cooperation, American Association of Community and Junior Colleges, 1979.
3.   Toombs, W., & Croyle, G. E. *A client reaction analysis: Final report for the Lifelong Learning Center, Reading, PA.* University Park, PA: Pennsylvania State University, Center for the Study of Higher Education, 1977.
4.   Toombs, W. *A study of client reactions. Lifelong Learning Center, The Free Library of Philadelphia.* University Park, PA: Pennsylvania State University, Center for the Study of Higher Education, 1978.

5. Dyer, P. S. *Final report on the higher education library advisory service project.* Albany, NY: University of the State of New York, Regents External Degree Program, 1978.
6. Paltridge, J. G., Regan, M. C., & Terkla, D. G. *Mid-career change: Adult students in mid-career transitions and community support systems developed to meet their needs.* Washington, D.C.: U.S. Office of Education, Community Services and Continuing Education Branch, 1978.
7. Kordalewski, J. B., & Alamprese-Johnson, J. *Impacts of services: The Regional Learning Service, 1974–77.* Syracuse, NY: Regional Learning Service of Central New York, 1977.
8. Deniston, O. L. *Evaluation of disease control programs.* Washington, D.C.: U.S. Department of Health, Education and Welfare, Public Health Service, 1974.
9. Deniston, O. L. *Program planning for disease control programs.* Washington, D.C.: U.S. Department of Health, Education and Welfare, Public Health Service, 1974.
10. Cross, K. P., & Zusman, A. The needs of non-traditional learners and the responses of non-traditional programs. *An evaluative look at non-traditional education.* Washington, D.C.: National Institute of Education, 1979.
11. Schlossberg, N. K. *A framework for studying adults in transition.* Paper presented at Second National Invitational Conference on Statewide Educational Information and Counseling Services, Denver, CO, February 1979.

REFERENCES

Anderson, R., & Darkenwald, G. *Participation and persistence in American adult education.* New York: College Entrance Examination Board, 1979.
Arbeiter, S., Aslanian, C. B., Schmerbeck, R. A., & Brickell, H. M. *40 million Americans in career transition: The need for information.* New York: College Entrance Examination Board, 1978. (a)
Arbeiter, S., Aslanian, C. B., Schmerbeck, F. A., & Brickell, H. M. *Telephone counseling for home-based adults.* New York: College Entrance Examination Board, 1978. (b)
Aslanian, C. B., & Brickell, H. M. *Americans in transition: Life changes as reasons for adult learning.* New York: College Entrance Examination Board, 1980.
Backstrom, C. H., & Hursh, C. D. *Survey research.* Evanston, IL: Northwestern University Press, 1963.
Brickell, H. M., & Paul, R. H. Evaluation. In C. B. Aslanian & H. B. Schmelter (Eds.), *Adult access to education and new careers: A handbook for action.* New York: College Entrance Examination Board, 1980.
Campbell, D. T., & Stanley, J. C. *Experimental and quasi-experimental designs for research.* Chicago: Rand McNally, 1966.
Christoffel, P., Ehrlich, N., & Macy, F. U. *Federal programs authorizing educational and occupational information services.* New York: College Entrance Examination Board, 1978.
Commission on Non-Traditional Study. *Diversity by design.* San Francisco: Jossey-Bass, 1973.
Cross, K. P. *The missing link: Connecting adult learners to learning resources.* New York: College Entrance Examination Board, 1978.
Glover, R., & Gross, B. *Future needs and goals for adult learning 1980–2000.* New York: College Entrance Examination Board, 1979.
Gould, S. B., & Cross, K. P. (Eds.). *Explorations in non-traditional study.* San Francisco: Jossey-Bass, 1972.
Grotelueschen, A. D. Program evaluation. In A. B. Knox (Ed.), *Developing, administering, and evaluating adult education.* San Francisco: Jossey-Bass, 1980.

Houle, C. O. *The design of education.* San Francisco: Jossey-Bass, 1972.
Johnstone, J. W. C., & Rivera, R. J. *Volunteers for learning.* Chicago: Aldine Publishing Company, 1965.
Knox, A. B. What difference does it make? In A. B. Knox (Ed.), *New directions for continuing education: Assessing the impact of continuing education.* San Francisco: Jossey-Bass, 1979.
Porter, A. C., & Chibucos, I. R. Selecting analysis strategies. In G. O. Borich (Ed.), *Evaluating educational programs and products.* Englewood Cliffs, NJ: Educational Technology Press, 1974.
Taber, T. D., Walsh, J. T., & Cooke, R. A. Developing a community-based program for reducing the social impact of a plant closing. *The Journal of Applied Behavioral Science*, 1979, *15*, 133–155.